*Psychology and
nursing children*

Psychology Applied to Nursing series

Recent and forthcoming titles in the series

Psychology and Mental Health Nursing   *Derek Milne*
Psychology of Nursing Care   *Neil Niven and Jill Robinson*
Psychology and Nursing Children   *Jo Douglas*

Psychology and nursing children

Jo Douglas

Principal Clinical Psychologist, The Hospital for Sick Children, Great Ormond Street, London

Series Editor: Professor Dave Müller, Suffolk College
Consultant: Erica Joslyn, Suffolk College

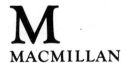

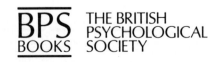

© Jo Douglas 1993

First published 1993 by
BPS Books (The British Psychological Society),
St. Andrews House, 48 Princess Road East, Leicester LE1 7DR
in association with
THE MACMILLAN PRESS LTD
Houndmills, Basingstoke, Hampshire RG21 2XS
and London
Companies and representatives
throughout the world

ISBN 0–333–56411–1
ISBN 0–333–56412–X

A catalogue record for this book is available
from the British Library

Typeset by Cambrian Typesetters, Frimley, Surrey
Printed in Hong Kong

Contents

List of tables and figures *vi*
Series Editor's Foreword *vii*
Acknowledgements *ix*

Introduction: Psychological skills for nurses *1*

Section One: Care of children in the community

1 Children and family life *19*
2 Primary health care of children in the community *50*
3 Children with special needs *71*
4 Children's behavioural and emotional problems *99*

Section Two: Caring for sick children

5 Caring for sick children in the community *129*
6 Care of sick children in hospital *152*
7 Care of the dying child *183*

Section Three: Caring for the carers

8 Be aware of yourself *201*

Postscript: Ethical issues in nursing *215*

References *221*

Suggested answers to exercises *231*

Index *237*

List of tables and figures

Table 1.1 A two-way classification of abuse with examples of major forms (Stratton, 1988) *35*

Table 1.2 Childhood Death Awareness Inventory (McCown, 1988) *46*

Table 2.1 Example of a multiple criteria screen for mother and toddler for emotional and behavioural problems (Nicol *et al.*, 1987) *56*

Table 2.2 Risk-factors checklist for abusing families (Browne and Stevenson, 1983) *57*

Table 2.3 Topics for a semi-structured interview *61*

Table 3.1 Variables significantly associated with outcome measures in univariate analyses for mothers (Sloper *et al.*, 1991) *92*

Table 3.2 Variables significantly associated with outcome measures in univariate analyses for fathers (Sloper *et al.*, 1991) *93*

Figure 3.1 Makaton signs *89*

Figure 3.2 Blissymbolics *90*

Figure 3.3 Two approaches to parent support *95*

Figure 4.1 Types of encopresis *101*

Table 4.1 Prevalence of drug use in 14 to 16-year-olds (Offord *et al.*, 1987) *102*

Table 4.2 Ontario Child Health Study (Offord *et al.*, 1987) *104*

Table 4.3 ABC chart *109*

Table 4.4 Formulation grid of contributing factors (Barker, 1988) *110*

Figure 4.2 Coercive behaviour of families of aggressive children *113*

Table 5.1 Analysis of family management behaviours (Deatrick and Knafl, 1990) *139*

Table 5.2 Seven topics chosen most frequently for discussion by parents of diabetic children (Moyer, 1989) *143*

Table 5.3 Areas of most concern to parents of diabetic children over the previous three months (Moyer, 1989) *143*

Table 8.1 Ways of Coping Scale (Folkman *et al.*, 1986) *208*

Series Editor's Foreword

This book series is designed for the nursing profession and those responsible for teaching nurses on both pre and post-registration programmes of study. The linking of the nursing curriculum with higher education and the implementation of Project 2000 has led to a radical revision of nurse education. Many nurses on pre-registration courses will be studying at degree level and will be gaining an academic qualification as well as entry to the nursing Register. These forward looking and exciting changes have led to the need to develop new reading material for nurses who wish to progress both academically and professionally.

This is equally true for those nurses post-registration who are committed to enhancing their qualifications' base. The expansion in higher education has led to a wide range of part-time degree courses for nurses as well as the linking of post-registration courses such as health visiting and district nursing with higher level academic qualifications. The introduction by the English National Board for Nursing, Midwifery and Health Visiting of the Higher Award for experienced professionals is an important step to facilitate continuing professional development for the nursing profession. This, in turn, has led to the need to bring together nursing and those disciplines akin to professional practice.

It has long been recognized that the study of psychology in applied contexts is of major importance both in learning to become a nurse and in moving towards becoming a reflective practitioner. Psychology as the scientific study of human behaviour provides a methodology through which individuals can evaluate the effectiveness of the provision of care within hospitals and the community. Psychology and nursing are both characterized by adopting a scientific and hence an empirical approach to the collection of information and using it to make informed decisions. The importance of research within the fields of psychology and nursing has led to psychologists and nurses working together both in terms of curriculum design and in carrying out research to help provide high standards of patient care.

All the books in the series are characterized by the emphasis placed on the critical examination of research evidence. Each volume aims to review current practice from a psychological perspective in the light of current research being undertaken by nurses as well as other professionals. The authors, in bringing together this information, all seek to offer recommendations to inform nursing practice not in a prescriptive way but in a way in which nurses themselves can evaluate their practice. All the texts are ideal for students studying psychology and nursing for the first time and are written at the appropriate level for inclusion on reading lists for students studying at diploma and degree level. At the same time, the applied research nature of the texts makes them invaluable as a source to support nurses gaining further qualifications as part of their professional development.

The texts are contemporary, derived from a strong research base and written by authors with considerble experience of teaching nurses and working with them professionally. I hope that you enjoy this volume in the serics and are attracted to the related texts which, taken together, provide nurses with a resource base from which to study psychology as applied to nursing.

Professor Dave Müller   *24 January 1993*
Suffolk College, Ipswich

Acknowledgements

I would like to dedicate this book to my family: my parents, Hywel and Dorothy Francis, my husband Robin and my two daughters, Alexandra and Amanda.

I would also like to thank the nursing staff and the patients of the Hospital for Sick Children, and in particular, Angela Wright, Senior Nurse Tutor, Richard Lansdown, Consultant Psychologist, and Bryan Lask, Consultant Psychiatrist, for their comments on the earlier drafts of the text. I would also like to thank Alexandra and Amanda for their delightful drawings; Hywel Francis for his amusing cartoons; and Dawn Sedgwick and pupils from Murrayfield Primary School, Ipswich, for drawings in Chapter 1.

Introduction: Psychological skills for nurses

The developmental context

Nursing children requires an understanding not only of their illnesses and medical conditions, but also of the social, psychological, and developmental influences that affect them. Children are not just small adults; they have special and changing requirements as they grow, and they make varying demands at different stages of their lives. Taking into account the child's age or stage of development, however, is not sufficient in recognizing the special requirements of nursing children, which involves understanding how the experiences in children's lives affect their ability to cope with illness and treatment, and how experiences around illness affect their future development and adult lives.

When considering the long- or short-term treatment of children, nurses need to be aware that each child is an individual with a personal trajectory of development. Their individual differences should be an integral part of nursing management, as they are unlikely to correlate simply with chronological age. It is important to remember that ill children are normal children with an illness. Being ill is part of their learning experience, and they can adapt to it, fight it, give up, or reject it. The problems faced by ill children need to be understood in terms of models that recognize the potential difficulties and coping resources of healthy families and children, not just those emphasizing psycho-pathology and malfunction (Eiser, 1990b).

Special features of paediatric nursing

Children differ from adult patients in their need for health care and support. The essential difference has been the developing awareness by nurses of the importance of families in the care of both ill and healthy children. The psycho-social context of illness in children cannot and should not be ignored. Children are dependent on their parents or carers for their health and safety for most of their childhood. They

1

carry no responsibility for this, particularly in their early years. They are also vulnerable to different types of illness with varying frequency from adults. They have a different understanding about illness and their bodies at different ages, and when young, are unable to report pain or symptoms in the same way as adults. As they grow older they need to learn treatment compliance and their nursing care requirements change.

The need for health education

Because parents carry most of the responsibility for the health of their child, in the early years the focus of health education for the baby and young child is geared towards the parents. Health surveillance checks, immunization programmes, and campaigns on health and safety in the home are all directed at parents, but the outcome of such programmes is the health of the child.

As children grow, it is necessary to direct their growing awareness and abilities so that they will begin to take responsibility for their own health, for example road safety, safety in the home, care of the teeth and diet awareness. Later, the issues of personal safety – safe sexual practices, drugs, smoking, and alcohol – all become high priority. Nurses have a significant role in ensuring that health education reaches all sections of the community and that families understand and can use the information for the health of their children.

Developmental changes in the incidence of illness

As they grow older, children experience different types of illnesses and accidents. Children between one and four have high rates of accidental poisoning; those between five and nine have high rates of pedestrian accidents; and older children have high rates of accidents involving recreational equipment (Eiser, 1990b). In particular, the reporting of children's accidents by parents should be considered in the context of development and abilities so that any form of child abuse can be accurately identified.

In regard to common childhood illnesses, the primary age range is particularly exposed to infectious diseases at school, such as chicken-pox, mumps, measles, and whooping cough. Common problems, such as colds and catarrh may have far-reaching effects in young children, who can suffer repeated otitus media and consequent intermittent hearing loss, which in turn can affect language development. Nurses need to be aware of the impact of childhood illnesses on the rapidly growing and developing child.

How children understand illness

Children's beliefs about illness and how the body works are part of their social, cultural, and learning background. Children require explanations that are appropriate to their level of conceptual understanding; the language and the methods of communication used need to fit the child's age, ability, and experience (Carey, 1985). For example, using pictures and playing with medically related toys like doctors' kits are often more appropriate with younger children than words. Nurses should try to understand attitudes within the child's family and culture so that information can be integrated with previous knowledge, and is provided in a sensitive and accessible form.

Reporting symptoms and pain

Children's ability to report symptoms depends on their language skills. Infants and young children express pain or illness through crying; they are unable to describe in words the type of pain or the feelings of illness they are experiencing. Parents and nursing staff need to guess by observing the child's non-verbal signals and physical signs how they are feeling. Gradually, children learn how to report their physical sensations to adults, but this can be affected by how these communications are received. Children are particularly vulnerable to adult responses as they are totally dependent on them for care and support. The adults may over-react, or may not respond to the child's statements and demands; they may not believe the child, or may consider them to be making an unnecessary fuss. The children may not report symptoms because of fears about what might happen to them, or that it might make their parents or the nurses angry. Alternatively, parents or nurses may actively encourage the expression of distress or pain, and at times there may be some specific gains of attention or special comforting that are associated with this. Nurses should observe carefully the impact of their response on the child and be cautious about interpreting the child's behaviour. The development of a relationship with a child is crucial in understanding their behaviour and for being sensitive to the non-verbal signals.

Treatment of illness and treatment compliance

At home, parents carry most of the responsibility for their children's medication or other ongoing treatment requirements. The instructions and the effort therefore has to be directed initially at them, and their co-operation is vital. They may need help in gaining treatment compliance from their child, and as the child grows older, may need help in handing over the responsibility for treatment compliance; for

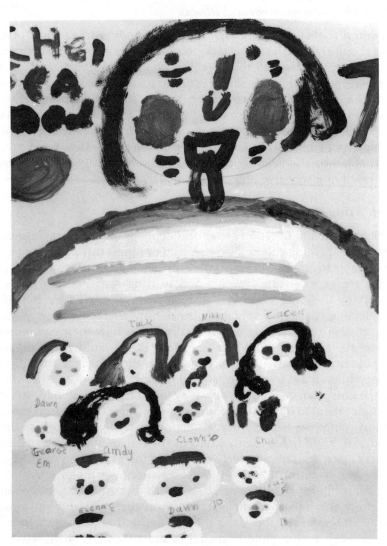

This picture was painted by an 8-year-old Jewish girl who nearly died from septic shock. When she recovered she decided to paint her experience. She started by painting a rainbow; she then asked the playleader what God looked like. The playleader said that 'God looks different to different people; what do you think he looks like?' Chelsea then painted white and blue stripes under the rainbow to show God as 'light'. She then painted the nurses on the ward and all of the children underneath, and finally painted a picture of herself on top of the rainbow with her tongue sticking out.

example, working with families to help ill adolescents take on their own health management in the context of increasing independence can be a significant area of preventative work.

Growth and changing requirements

Children rapidly grow and change, and their treatment requirements and nursing care should grow and change with them: the type of care on the ward required for a pre-school child and an adolescent are very different. The type of support and help required by parents with children of different ages is also very different. Because families also change and grow, the effects of chronic illness on siblings and on the developmental stages of family life may need to be considered.

The influence of family relationships

Children's experiences within the family will have a considerable effect on their health and on their social and emotional development. Problems in the parents', or the parent–child relationship, or rivalry with siblings can affect ill children as much as well children. The family's communication pattern, alliances, and conflicts all have a considerable effect on children's psychological development. When there is an ill child, there is another source of stress in family life with which family members must cope. Their way of coping may in turn affect the course of the child's illness, and his or her ability to cope with symptoms and treatment. Emotional and behavioural problems in the child as a result of disturbed family relationships can severely disrupt nursing and medical care. Nurses may feel that these problems are interfering with the task of nursing, but these problems are an integral part of caring for the whole child and need to be addressed.

The sharing of feelings and crises are important in the family adaptation and management of chronic or acute illness. Many families cope very well with caring for an ill child, and their abilities to do so may be enhanced by the experience. Nurses should be aware of such families, and try to learn from them in order to better support families who do not manage so well.

Enhancing parents' skills: intervention in the community

Families that are under stress or demonstrate problems in general child care may or may not be seeking help, but when the primary health care team becomes aware of the potential problems for the child, intervention is often necessary. Because the family may initially reject outside help, the nurse's first goal is to form a relationship with the parents. Once the parents are able to be open about what is happening and how they are feeling, the nurse can begin to mobilize the parents' resources and abilities to cope.

Case study

Lee, aged four years, was in hospital for management of constipation and overflow after early operations for an imperforate anus. While on the ward nurses became concerned about his mother's reactions to him, having seen her hit him and tell him he was wicked for soiling his pants and never having seen her cuddle him. Contact with the local agencies indicated that concern had been expressed by his nursery teacher and social services about the mother's behaviour towards Lee, but no action had been taken. In hospital it was possible for the mother to tell nurses how difficult Lee was to manage and how she had been told he was an aggressive boy who would always be bad. Once she could express her worries it was possible to arrange for her to receive some help and counselling from the health visitor and social worker.

The aim of intervention is not to foster a dependent relationship between the parents and the nurse, but to enable the parents to take responsibility for change, and to be strengthened in the task of parenting. The building up of confidence and skills is an essential component of this task: the parents need to be praised and encouraged in their efforts to manage the situation; they need to be prompted to find alternative ways of coping with the child. Nurses can draw out the parents' inner resources to solve their problems. Suggestions or giving advice should occur only when it is wanted and can be accepted and used. At times, parents may not have the emotional resources to cope with the problems of parenting and, when the nurse detects the possibility of little or no change, then liaison with other services in the community to provide support will be necessary.

Forming a therapeutic relationship

The basis of a good therapeutic relationship is to show 'unconditional positive regard' towards the parent or child (Rogers, 1951). This means that the client feels accepted and liked no matter what he or she says or does. When a client feels this they may be better able to share their feelings without fear of criticism. Rapport is important, but this does not necessarily imply informality. Empathy, sensitivity, and warmth are the essential ingredients. Empathy is the ability to experience others' feelings together with an ability to communicate understanding of those feelings. A sensitive nurse will be able to identify the differences in parents between visits or between what a parent is saying and feeling. Emotional warmth creates an accepting and caring attitude that families and children will respond to and feel they can trust. For these therapeutic skills to develop and be used, nurses must be aware of their own attitudes and feelings. For example, if the nurse feels angry with or rejected by a family, then their feelings may interfere with their ability to communicate. These skills require practice and nurses need to recognise the importance of this 'therapeutic role' rather than relying only on their natural social skills.

Types of communication

When talking to a family, the nurse should take account of:

- body language (facial expression, posture, and eye contact);
- what is said (words used, how sentences are phrased; speed, intonation, pitch, and loudness of voice);
- emotions and feelings.

Body language (facial expression, posture and eye contact)

Body language is a form of non-verbal communication that is very important. Nurses need to be conscious of the messages they are sending as well as what is being received. For instance, eye contact can be revealing. Because the British tend to look more at people they like, if eye contact is not made repeatedly during a conversation, it may be interpreted as disinterest, dislike, anger, or a fear of exposure. In fact, it may be due to shyness, preoccupation, or depression. There are significant cultural differences in the amount of eye contact that is felt to be permissible. Some find eye contact too aggressive and feel it is impolite to look directly at the person to whom they are talking.

Facial expression is also important. While smiling makes people feel more at ease, some people cover up their true feelings by smiling inappropriately. It is therefore important to match the person's facial expression with what they are saying, and be aware of discrepancies. Again, cross cultural differences in facial expressiveness can be misinterpreted. Sometimes a thoughtful expression can appear cross or worried, and this can be misleading. The nurse's facial expression should indicate interest. If the child or parent is sad or unhappy, obviously the nurse should not be cheerfully smiling. Nodding and making supportive noises will prompt the talker to continue. This 'active listening' requires effort and practice (Hyland and Donaldson, 1989).

Posture, how people sit, whether they fidget, and how close they stand will also give clues about feelings and emotions. For example, the difference in posture between a depressed and an anxious person is usually very noticeable.

Touching can also be helpful, particularly if a parent or child is showing distress. If tears get in the way of talking about a problem, then silence and a gentle touch on the arm by the nurse can indicate empathy.

Activity
Role play is a very useful way of learning how to communicate effectively and also how to observe clients' behaviour. A video recording of the event will give you feedback on how you appear to others while trying to be empathic. Plan three scenes with one very anxious mother who talks continuously about her child's asthma, a mother who pretends that everything is fine while coping with a child who has cerebral palsy, and a mother who is depressed about her child's soiling. Try role playing these three situations with a fellow student.

Talking with families and children

Talking with parents and children is the main way to find out what is happening, how they are feeling or thinking, and what information and help is required. Questioning can either help a person to open up, or make them frightened, angry, or resentful. Nobody likes to be interrogated, and so the style and tone of questioning is important. The best approach is to be gentle and sympathetic, while observing closely the effect of questions on the parents and child.

Open and closed questions

The type of question asked will encourage either full, informative answers, or just a precise answer and no more. So-called 'closed questions' can usually be answered by 'yes' or 'no' and are used to gain factual information in a precise way, e.g. 'Are you feeling better today?' 'Open questions' are more likely to encourage the speaker to volunteer extra information, e.g. 'How are you feeling today?' In general, it is better to use open questions.

Structuring the discussion

The way in which the discussion is structured will also affect the type and amount of information given and received. 'Directive questioning' should be used when necessary information is required, for example in a diagnostic setting or when there is limited time, e.g. 'How many times did he wake last night?' It can be very thorough, and may initiate an exploratory discussion later on. 'Non-directive' questioning is used when general areas of information are sought. Here, the lead is taken from the parent's or child's comments. By asking them to expand on their comments, the nurse can find out what is important to them, e.g. 'You say he's been naughty today, can you tell me more about that?'

'Reflecting back' what has just been said is also a way of prompting further discussion and of expressing empathy. It is also a good way of finding out whether what has just been said has been understood. For example, a mother may say 'Johnny didn't sleep at all last night, and I feel terrible', to which the nurse could reflect back, 'You must feel exhausted, after so little sleep'.

Expressing emotions

A lot of the support offered by the nurse involves recognising the parents' feelings – whether this is the stress of looking after a dying child, the problems of an overactive pre-schooler, or coping with a handicapped adolescent. Some people have great difficulty expressing their feelings; others do not really understand how they feel; others will say things are going well when in fact they are feeling very stressed. In the latter case, there will be a discrepancy between what is said and the behaviour. A mother may say she is feeling fine, but not make eye contact, or fidget and pick anxiously at her fingers.

Working with parents

The ability to transmit information efficiently and effectively is a complex skill, and all too often professionals do not have the opportunity to learn how to do it. Knowledge given out by an expert can be misused or rejected, even though it is correct and well founded. The 'expert' may feel a good job has been done, without realizing how ineffective the communication in fact has been. The community nurse, however, is in a prime position to interface between the needs of parents and child health care information, just as the hospital-based nurse is often called on by parents to interpret medical information.

Fitting advice into a framework that can be understood and used is as important as the advice itself: giving information is a waste of time unless it is heard correctly and can be used. All too often parents or children are given information that they do not remember, do not understand, or reject because it does not fit in with their own views. In many areas of child care, parents hold certain views and opinions that need to be taken into consideration when new information is being offered. The health professional should work with the parents to develop and enhance good child care skills, rather than act as the 'expert' giving out factual information on good parenting.

Models of consultation

The nurse's approach should vary according to the problem being discussed: at times a parent may request urgent and direct practical nursing help, while at other times they may want to discuss their child's behaviour, illness, or development. Cunningham and Davis (1985) have described three models of consultation.

The expert model

Here, the professional rather than the patient takes control of all decision making. Information is selected that is considered relevant to the patient's needs, and that the professional considers important. This is a very 'medical' approach to consultation, where the health professional has special diagnostic or treatment skills that are offered to the patient in a time-limited manner. Parents often feel dependent on the professional and take little responsibility for their own decisions. They may feel incompetent and undermined in their parenting role, for example that they have failed their child or that the problem is their fault. Because no real dialogue is established, they often fail to ask questions, feel overwhelmed, and do not reveal how little they have understood. The outcome is that parents either become very dependent on the professional's advice, or they feel dissatisfied and fail to carry out the advice or suggestions.

The transplant model

Here, the professional tries to 'transplant' his or her skills on to the parents, but often retains control of the decision-making process. Many health professionals working with parents and children who have behavioural and emotional problems adopt this approach as they recognize it is the parents who will carry out the changes, and so they need to feel competent and able. This approach is dependent on a good working relationship in which communication and parental satisfaction are high.

When parents seek advice on how to cope with their child, the community nurse may need to facilitate the skills the parents already have. Encouraging the parents' ability to think of alternatives, or of the outcome of their existing views, can often help them to realize they may not be correct. The best way to help is to enable parents to think

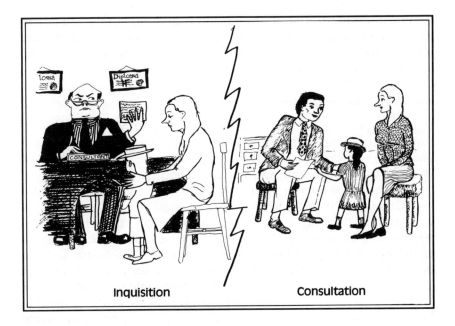

Inquisition | Consultation

up the answer themselves, or to present the information in such a way that they think they thought of it. On the ward, parents may need to be taught nursing procedures to carry out at home, and although these may seem simple and straightforward to the nurse, they may be frightening or upsetting to the parents. It is important to remember that each family is different. The nurse must understand the family and its cultural and social context before trying to intervene and effect any change in the family pattern of behaviour. Time is needed to listen to and gain the trust of the family, and for advice or instructions to be tailored to their needs.

The consumer model

The role of the health professional in this model is to listen and to understand the parents' views and expectations, and to offer a range of alternatives, options, and information. The professional thus becomes a resource and a route to information, someone to help balance the alternatives and to widen the options available. This approach is often used when working with parents who have handicapped children, or with children who have chronic medical conditions and who are being cared for at home. The nurse should acknowledge that the parents know more about the situation than anyone else. Their knowledge may be so detailed in a particular field of child health care that it surpasses that of most health professionals. This should be acknowledged and valued. There should be an open exchange of information and a sharing in decision-making. The professional should not attain power just by status and title, but should be effective in delivering a service, and in establishing a negotiating process. Nurses should always be prepared to learn from parents' and children's experiences.

Children's developmental needs

If the purpose of the community health practitioner's visits is to support the parents in their parenting role, then nurses need to have a good working knowledge of the development and problems of children; how to play with and talk to different age groups, the types of toys and activities they enjoy, how to make and provide play materials, are all things with which parents may require help (Newson and Newson, 1979). Being up to date with the recent crazes in toys and television programmes is one way in which nurses can start to communicate with children and parents. Similarly, the nurse needs to be aware of the importance of talking to and with young children so that parents are encouraged to extend their child's vocabulary and language development. Nurses will be involved in nursing or supporting children with varying special needs, including behavioural, intellectual and physical disabilities (see Chapter 3).

Issues of discipline and control are also very important. The nurse needs to be aware of effective methods and strategies for helping parents cope with behaviour problems, but must also be able to apply this knowledge in the context of their relationship with, and the needs of, the parents. Helping parents to find the right technique and approach for them is far more effective than telling them what to do (see Chapter 4).

Giving information

Information should be given in the context of the listener's knowledge and experience. Determining if parents or children are likely to understand what has been said, and their emotional reactions, are both important. Giving information is not just stating simple facts: it should be balanced with questioning of the parent or child so that it fits in to their understanding. There are three main aims in providing information.

☐ Helping people to understand what they have been told
Basic information and instructions should be simple and straightforward using words that the parent or child can understand. The nurse should anticipate any areas of misunderstanding, and try to find out what the parent or child does understand by sensitive questioning. If asked outright, 'Do you understand?' most people will say 'yes', despite being unsure. Pictures, books, diagrams, and models can all help. On the

other hand, some parents and children are very knowledgeable about their illness or condition, especially if they have had frequent admissions to hospital. They may simply want more detail and require extensive information.

Make sure the parent or child is paying attention. If discussion is in the home, then the parent should be asked to sit down to talk. The television, radio, or stereo should be switched off, or go to a quieter area. If a mother has a young child making demands on her during the discussion, then she should be given time to meet the needs of the child before continuing.

Nurses should be aware of the parent's or child's emotional state while talking, and also of their emotional reaction to the information. An anxious or depressed parent may readily misperceive information, or may be too preoccupied with their own thoughts to listen properly. They may need more time and space to hear what is being discussed. Repeat what is said several times and in different ways so that all the problems can be clarified.

Make sure the child understands what is happening. It may be appropriate first to discuss with the parents what to tell the child and how to tell them, and then either to encourage the parent to tell the child in front of you, or to offer to tell the child yourself. The child's development level and the level of understanding are important. Talking with children is a skill and requires practice; the nurse's aim should be to allow a discussion to develop, with the child asking questions rather than simply talking at the child.

Exercise

Consider a situation in which two children, one aged five and one aged twelve have just been diagnosed as having leukaemia. Who do you think should tell the child? How could this be phrased best for each child's developmental level? Find out how colleagues and senior staff have talked about this with parents and children. What techniques could be used to support giving this information to the child? Think about models, drawings or analogies that could be used to aid understanding of the disease.

☐ Helping people to remember what they have been told

Often, we understand information at the time it is told to us, but it can be difficult to recall it later on. People often remember the first and the last things said, and forget the middle, and so presentation is important. Also, the more information presented at one time, the more that will be forgotten. It can be helpful to write down the information so the family can refer to it later. It should be organized in a list form, be numbered sequentially, and be legible. Ask the family where they are going to keep the list. Do not forget to write down your own name, where you can be contacted, and the telephone number. Families often forget the names of professionals and then feel too embarrassed to ask the next time they see you. Think about how you would remember a lot of new information that is unfamiliar and learn to slow the pace and provide guides to remembering.

☐ Helping people to accept what they have been told

People often reject information that is threatening or if they do not want to do as they are told. For example, parents may deny that their child is ill, handicapped, or has been abused. This is very threatening information; it may reflect on their treatment of the child, or expose feelings of guilt and blame. Nurses must be very sensitive and careful when giving this type of information, or it will be met with outright denial, aggression, or anger.

Of course, a warm, supportive, and trusting relationship is necessary before any disclosure is made. Gentle prompting to find out how much family members know or suspect is part of the process. They also need to be ready to receive the information, in a questioning frame of mind, wanting to find out more, and prepared for bad news. Sometimes parents want news, but not bad news. It can be helpful to prompt them into thinking about possible answers, including threatening information. If parents can come to the correct conclusion themselves, even if this is threatening, they are far more likely to believe it. Otherwise they will accept information only if it is consistent with their beliefs. Repeated visits and several attempts to move parents' thoughts towards the problem may be necessary.

Some parents or children refuse to accept information because they do not want to do what is asked. This may be because they don't believe what has been said – that it is too threatening; that you are an outsider and do not understand them – or they can't be bothered. Sometimes underlying factors in the family relationship prevent compliance; a disturbed marital relationship, for example, can prevent parents working together to manage their child's behaviour problem. Or a child may refuse to take medication because it is part of a general battle with the mother about control. Or a mother may refuse to carry out instructions about how to feed her baby because they conflict with her own mother's instructions. The nurse needs to be credible to the family, and to be able to discuss clearly the reasons why they should comply, and to be persuasive, not condescending, angry or patronizing.

Partnerships for child care

Safeguarding the welfare of the child is one of the main principles of the Children Act (1989). In order to achieve this aim, the Act stresses the importance of developing a working partnership with the child's family as the most effective way of providing help to families with child care and child rearing problems (White *et al.*, 1990). This partnership requires not only listening to parents and taking their concerns and priorities seriously but also involves recognizing that just because a parent does not always have the skills or the patience to care for a child properly, this does not mean they do not care about the child.

The Act is intended to make the law relating to children more appropriate to their needs in recognizing that children coping with either multiple disabilites or children from troubled families do not have needs which can be neatly compartmentalized into health, education and social support. The Act is designed to build the relationship between the providers of services for children and families and the families who use these services. The main difficulty with this kind of partnership is that whereas in most partnerships the partners have positively chosen to work together, here neither partner may feel they have much option. Parents may feel pressured by the belief that the alternative to co-operation is to have help formally imposed or, at worst, to have their children taken away from the family home. Partnerships in these circumstances will not simply happen. They need to be worked at and must be based on an honest, clear, mutual understanding of what is to be achieved and how.

The 1989 Act extends the value of partnerships to include working relationships between different agencies and directs the various agencies to consult each other, keep each other informed, and to co-operate to achieve common goals. The Act requires that appropriate packages of services involving different agencies should be developed in partnership with the family following discussions with the child.

Within the Act, health professionals have a duty to co-operate with social services departments. In particular, child care nurses, nurses working in accident and emergency departments, and community nurses, who come into contact with children as a consequence of their practice, have a responsibility to participate in the design and implementation of services for the care of children. In addition, nurses are in the valuable position of possibly being the first to be able to alert others to the position of a child in need.

Summary

The psychological care of children and their families by nurses demands that each child and parent is understood and supported as a unique individual. A non-judgmental attitude from the nurse, and an ability to enhance and encourage the best coping qualities in the family are necessary. A respect for individuality, and an ability to show empathy, sensitivity, and warmth are required by all nurses to create a supportive and therapeutic relationship. Communication with parents and children is the basis of this work and nurses need to learn effectively how to provide supportive counselling with constructive advice and information.

There are large gaps in our knowledge and understanding of children's psychological growth and development, as well as the psychology of dealing with children's illness. This book introduces the basic concepts in the psychological care of children and families, and provides research-based findings relevant to nursing practice. As this touches only the surface of knowledge in this area, further in-depth reading will be necessary and references are given. Some research findings are described in detail in order to provide an introduction to, and an illustration of, the type of experimental and research-based approaches being used at present.

Further reading

Cunningham, C. C. and Davis, H. (1985) *Working with Parents: Frameworks for Collaboration*. Milton Keynes, Open University Press.

SECTION ONE

Care of children in the community

1 *Children and family life*

Introduction

Children experience immense differences in their home and family lives. The stereotypical mother and father, their two children, plus a cat and a dog is no longer relevant to today's society. Many children now live in single-parent families. In 1987, 14 per cent of families with dependent children had only one parent; this was double the figure for 1971. Births outside marriage rose from 11 per cent in 1979 to 27 per cent in 1989. According to the Central Statistical Office, in 1989, 36 per cent of marriages were re-marriages, while the number of women cohabiting trebled between 1979 and 1988.

Many children have step-parents or intermittent substitute parents. Children may be raised by nannies, childminders or grandparents. They may live in group-care settings or have foster or adoptive parents. They may be loved, nurtured, and well cared for – or rejected, abused, and abandoned. They may be stimulated and played with – or neglected and ignored. They may come from a background of wealth and comfort – or of stress and poverty. All of these factors play a part in the children's social and emotional development, and help to determine how they respond to others, make relationships, and grow into caring adults, who perhaps will in turn become parents.

Children are vulnerable members of our society. In the past they have been variously treated as their parents' possessions, an unwanted drain on family resources, or a potential labour source rather than as individuals with rights and expectations for a future of their own.

More recently, children in Western society have been recognized as having their own rights. Although the law now offers some safeguards, old attitudes die hard, and many of the issues around children's rights are still controversial. For example, the right to go to school and receive an education is now well recognized in this country, but how much right does a child have in a divorce settlement in saying which parent they would prefer to live with?

There are a number of significant influences in children's family lives that will be reflected in their later development. Many of these will influence the health professional's role and ability to care for the children when ill.

Attachment

The concept of attachment is one way of describing the closeness-seeking and care-eliciting behaviour of children to caring adults. In 1959, H. F. Harlow found that baby monkeys spent more time cuddling a soft material-covered substitute mother than a wire-mesh substitute mother complete with feeding teats. John Bowlby developed these ideas further into the 'attachment theory'. This has given rise to a model of human behaviour that has stimulated an enormous amount of research into children's relationships with their parents and other significant adults and has had a great effect on nursing practice.

By careful observation in controlled settings, Ainsworth *et al.* (1978) attempted to categorize the different types of attachment behaviour that children show. In the 'strange situation' experiments, one-year-old infants and their mothers were observed in various combinations of the child with and without the mother and a stranger. Ainsworth found there are marked differences in how children react and has attempted to classify them. Most infants, 60 to 65 per cent, are clearly (or 'securely') attached to their mothers. When placed in a strange situation they want to be close to her, but will gradually start to explore the new surroundings from a safe base. If left alone in a strange setting for a short time the children become very clingy when the mother reappears. The mothers of such children tend to be responsive and sensitive to their children's needs, and so encourage attachment.

About 20 per cent of infants show little upset both at the absence of the parent and when reunited. They tend to avoid interacting with their mother, and are thus referred to as 'avoidantly' attached children. The mothers are often insensitive to their children's signals; they rarely have close physical contact, and are often angry and irritable.

Approximately 10 to 15 per cent of infants, the 'ambivalently attached', show frequent intense distress whether the mother is present or absent. They either lack interest in being close to the mother, or show ambivalence by intermittently seeking closeness and then angrily rejecting her. Mothers of such children are often insensitive and awkward in their interaction with the child; while not very affectionate, they are not as rejecting as avoidant mothers. Nurses will frequently observe the reactions of infants to separation from their parents and may need to intervene at times to aid a mother's understanding of her child's behaviour.

An attachment is a special affectionate link that one person makes to another that endures over time and distance, and characterizes most relationships between children and their parents. Attachments take time to form and develop through experience with the other person. The process of attachment occurs both from the baby to the parent(s)

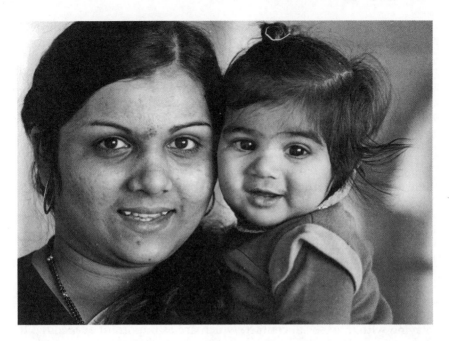

© Camilla Jessel and Action for Sick Children. Reproduced by permission.

or main caregiver, and from the parent(s) or main caregiver to the baby. Infants frequently become attached to nurses who have cared for them for long periods and equally nurses become attached to the children.

Research has demonstrated that the quality of the caregiver's behaviour towards a six-month-old child will affect the child's later attachment behaviour; it will also influence the caregiver's behaviour towards the child at age two years, and even the child's behaviour towards a sibling three years later (Sroufe, 1985). Infants with secure attachments to their caregiver at 12 to 18 months are less likely to show high dependency on that caregiver when playing with other children and with adults at four and five years of age. Children who are insecurely attached are more likely to have less positive attitudes to their peer group, and also to have behavioural and social difficulties (Sroufe and Fleeson, 1988).

Activity
Observe three children on the ward: a six-month-old, a two-year-old, and a four-year-old. Observe the separation behaviours these children show when their parent(s) leave the ward for a meal and how both the parent and child prepare for and manage the separation. Do the parents tell the child

that they are leaving or do they leave quickly with no warning? Do the parents ask a nurse to sit and amuse their child while they leave? Does the child show distress? Can the child be distracted and amused? Does the child anticipate the parents leaving and start to cling or ask them not to go? Do the parents show distress at leaving?

The baby's need for attachment

Babies who do not receive personal attention, stimulation, and caring tend to show marked delays in thinking, talking, and social development. The most important aspect of this marked deprivation is its long-term nature; continuous exposure to severe deprivation and adversity seriously impairs the child's normal social and intellectual development. Only if the environment can be altered is there a chance of decreasing the effects of deprivation.

Babies form attachments in order to ensure they receive the care and attention needed for survival. This does not mean they form attachments only to those who feed them: babies also need cuddling, playing with, and social contact, which are as important as feeding. It does not have to be the mother to whom the baby bonds, although she is the person most likely to fulfil the function of caregiver. Babies make different attachments to different people in their lives: fathers, grandparents, nannies, and child-minders can all become very important people to the baby (Lewis, 1986). The main feature of the baby–adult relationship is that the carer should spend 'quality' time giving personal attention over a prolonged period to the baby, so that they get to know each other, and understand each others' signals and communications. The carer and baby both require time and experience with each other to develop a reciprocal awareness so that they are in tune with each others' needs and reactions.

Nurses need to understand the process of attachment and its effect on the child's behaviour and future emotional development. Being cared for by many different carers can be difficult for babies and young children experiencing long stays in hospital during their early years. For some children, hospital is home during their first few years of life. Such children present a special problem for nursing staff, as they form attachments to staff who leave or must change shifts. If the parents are unable to visit regularly or frequently enough during such long stays, the child's early attachments will be to the nurses. Unfortunately, while the person in charge of the ward may be the most constant person in the child's life, she may also be the person who can spend the least time with the child.

The many different hospital staff and visitors mean that the long-stay child receives fleeting social contact with a lot of strangers, many of whom may pat or pick the child up, not realizing the effect this may have on the child's long-term social development. Nurses may need to consider limiting the number of indiscriminate social contacts a long stay child has and deliberately choose two or three staff as attachment figures, who carry a special responsibility for the psychological welfare of the child. If possible, the parents should be encouraged to give their child quality time when they visit, ensuring that the child makes a special attachment to them that is enduring over and beyond the length of the child's stay in hospital.

Case study

Gurpal, aged 2 years, who had been in hospital for a year, was starting to show socially precocious and difficult behaviour. He would race up to anyone entering the ward and want to be picked up. He was demanding of attention from nursing staff, intrusive to other children's privacy and their families, and disobedient. Observation of his social contacts in the course of an hour revealed continual interruption of his play by staff and visitors patting him, asking him questions and greeting him. Nurses had to learn to respect his privacy and play, to ask visitors not to pick him up and to allocate three main staff to be his main carers and develop consistent management of his behaviour.

Exercise

Consider the emotional needs of two one-year-old children in hospital, one for a short stay of two days, and the other for an indefinite period of several months. Identify the different roles the nurse needs to play for the two children, and specify the optimal nursing care and psychological support for each child and its parents.

The parent's need for attachment to the baby

The issues around early attachment have affected nursing practice considerably during the past 20 years. In the mid-1970s, research indicated that if mothers and their newborn babies were separated after birth there could be later problems in the mother–child relationship (Klaus and Kennell, 1976). This had great implications for the care of mother and newborn baby, encouraging medical and nursing practice to facilitate contact in the early hours and days of the baby's life. Later research indicated that the concern generated was rather exaggerated; there does not appear to be a short critical time for human mothers and babies to bond, as there is in many other animal species. The change in hospital practice, however, has been for the better as it has recognized the great importance of this early period (Sluckin *et al.*, 1983).

This does not deny the fact that the parents need time to develop an attachment to their baby. Many first time mothers feel distressed when they do not immediately feel a surge of love and affection for their newborn baby, which can take time to develop as mothers get to know their babies, and vice versa. Nurses can play an important role in helping the new mother understand her baby. When new mothers are given information by nurses about the social abilities of their babies and how to communicate with them, they become more attuned and are able to make an attachment more easily.

A controlled research study that demonstrated an assessment of neonatal behaviour to new mothers and fathers showed there was a positive effect on the quality of interaction between the parents and their babies as they became more aware of their new baby's behaviour. There was an increase in the experimental group, compared to the control group, in parents' smiling, touching, vocalizing, positioning, and responsiveness (Beale, 1989). However, controversy has developed over the lack of positive long-term implications of early interventions on attachment. Many of the studies that have attempted to positively intervene with high-risk infants and their parents have failed to demonstrate long term effects (Belsky, 1985).

Nurses can have an important role in making direct observations on parent–infant interaction during the neonatal period. Beale (1991) has emphasized the need for nurses to develop and use valid and reliable measurement tools that relate to a clear definition of attachment that includes the level of mutual reciprocal interchange and affection between the parent and infant. Parents who can identify distinct characteristics of their baby and who are able to respond to their baby's cries are showing attachment. This can be monitored by interview as well as by direct observation.

Separation

Once the baby or young child has formed attachments to carers, the issue of separation becomes important. As they grow up, all children need to learn how to separate from their parents and others. Sometimes these separations are carefully planned and anticipated, but at other times they may be abrupt and possibly traumatic, for example if the mother or child is taken to hospital urgently.

Children begin to show separation anxiety at about eight months, which is also the time they start to show a wariness of strangers. Their anxiety peaks at between 12 and 18 months. Many parents naturally introduce gradual and brief separations toward the end of the second year in order to prepare the child for playgroup and playing with friends. When young children experience predictable, enjoyable, and short separations, they learn what to expect and how to manage their anxiety. When they are familiar with the environment in which they are being left, and also with the people who are to look after them while the parent is absent, then anxiety is minimized. Unpredictable separations, however, in which the child is taken to a new place with unfamiliar people can be very frightening, even for a child who has learned to separate well. Although an acute life event such as this may induce symptoms of anxiety and social withdrawal in the child, once he or she is back with the parents, the symptoms usually resolve in a few days; there do not appear to be any long-term effects (Rutter, 1981).

Observations of young children experiencing prolonged separations show they pass through a series of emotional reactions. The first is often protest, when the child will cry and not let anyone help. The second is despair, when the child may become quiet and apathetic. Finally, the child may become 'detached'. Unfortunately, the less demanding the child is when alone, the greater the intensity of the despair at separation. This can seem confusing to inexperienced staff, who feel relieved when a child stops crying, misinterpreting his or her quietness as acceptance of the situation. All nursing staff need to watch carefully for signs of withdrawal, apathy, and detachment in children left in hospital alone. A classic example of this has been seen recently in orphanages in Romania where very low staff levels and inadequate stimulation of the children led to children sitting passively rocking in their cots with no response to passing adults.

The impact of separation on the child is increased if there has been a poor-quality relationship with the parent (Rutter, 1985). A good parent–child relationship, therefore, provides some protection against the negative effects of separation. Knowledge of the parent–child relationship before long-term admission to hospital may be one way of understanding the effects of separation on the child, and of identifying how best to help the child and parents to cope. Parents may need clear guidelines on the necessity for visiting or being resident, the importance of playing with their child and being present during unpleasant procedures. Nurses can make parents feel important in the care of their child while in hospital by pointing out the child's reactions and positively linking the child's and parent's behaviour in a supportive manner.

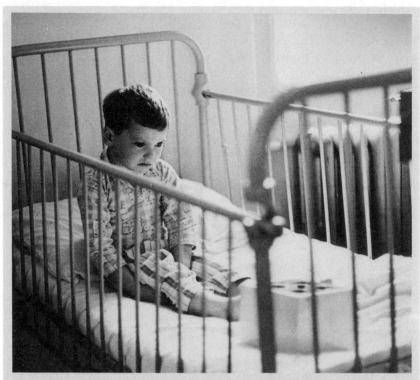

© Camilla Jessel and Action for Sick Children. Reproduced by permission.

Exercise
This photograph is what we don't want to see in hospital. How different is this from the ideal hospital environment for a young child? Think of four changes that could easily be made. (Suggested answers at end of book.)

Maternal deprivation

The concept of maternal deprivation was first raised by John Bowlby in the early 1950s. It was Bowlby's opinion that babies and young children must have a continuous, unbroken relationship with one person to make an attachment and to ensure healthy social and emotional development. Consequently, strong pressure was exerted on mothers to stay at home with their pre-school children rather than go out to work. It also affected parental visiting practices in hospitals, so that parents could stay all day rather than just attend at defined times, and mothers were encouraged to stay overnight with their children. In residential care facilities, fostering was encouraged rather the use of children's homes, so that children could make an attachment to consistent adults rather than the transient relationships made with residential staff in children's homes.

In the late 1960s and early 1970s, faced with new research evidence, Bowlby changed his views, stating that children need to make stable, long-term attachments, but that these need not be only to the mother. Today, it is generally agreed that mothers need not feel guilty about going out to work and arranging day-care facilities for their young children, as long as the care is of high quality, and the children can create attachments to the day-care staff (Rutter, 1981). This has implications for nursing practice of long stay children.

The quality of the attachment to the mother is an important factor in enabling the child to cope with separation. When securely attached, then no adverse effects of day-care are detectable; where the parent–child relationship is very poor, the quality of the child's attachment to the day-care staff may be very important emotionally, and help to compensate for problems at home. But it is important to keep in mind that the hospitalized child is not just experiencing an alternative care environment. The child is ill and may have to endure painful procedures that are traumatic. The needs of the child for the parent are therefore much more important.

Parenting

Families differ markedly in their parenting styles and in the amount of play and stimulation they offer their children. In assessing good

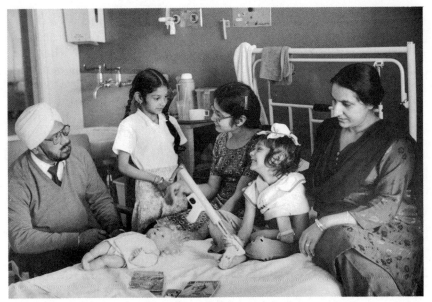

© Camilla Jessel and Action for Sick Children. Reproduced by permission.

parenting, many different aspects can be analyzed. Consider the love/ hostility aspects, for example, in which the parents may be very accepting and loving towards the child and provide an atmosphere of warmth and affection, compared to those who are rejecting and disapproving of their child, creating a cold, critical environment. Another aspect is control/autonomy: some parents are very rigid and strict in their control of their children, while others are permissive and set no limits.

The effects of these different parenting styles on children can be very marked, and will affect their personalities and behaviours throughout childhood, and even into adult life. Children raised in a loving and tolerant home are more likely to be sociable, have good self-esteem, and a positive view of themselves and others. In comparison, children who have had a loving but more controlled home environment may become more dependent and submissive. And children who are raised in hostile and rejecting homes may feel worthless, have problems relating to their own age group, and have difficulty with authority figures. Styles of parental authority fall into three categories:

- Authoritarian parents, who expect their children to obey them unquestioningly.
- Authoritative parents, who exert control over their children, but will reason and explain. Such parents value obedience and conformity, but also independence and self-direction.
- Permissive parents, who impose few regulations and adopt an accepting, non-evaluative role. (Baumrind, 1980)

The type of child-rearing and parenting that is established in a child's early years will strongly affect the parent–child relationship in adolescence. Where there are clear and rational limits, but where the child's view is accepted and incorporated, when possible, it can lay a good grounding for a considerate and caring relationship, with parent and child expressing mutual respect (Conger and Peterson, 1984). Nurses encounter many different parenting styles and need to care for children from varying home backgrounds. A considerate, sensitive, informative and consistent style of nursing will enable children to develop trust and demonstrate their feelings.

Maternal depression

Maternal depression can have a marked effect on the development of the child. Observations have demonstrated that depressed mothers make fewer links between their child's activities and the context of their behaviour. For example, if a child pointed to a bus, the mother who is not depressed might comment, 'Yes, that's just like the bus we went on yesterday to the shops.' This would enable the child to make the situation relevant to his or her own world. A depressed mother is not in tune with her child's thoughts and actions, and so the opportunities for the development of responsive and adaptive inter-actions is diminished (Mills *et al.*, 1985). A depressed mother may ignore the child's action, tell them to stop pointing or just say 'Yes' in a distracted and bored manner. Depressed mothers are preoccupied with their own thoughts; they are distracted and fail to initiate or respond to their child's cues. They also demonstrate more smacking and criticism of the child and less smiling and affectionate touching than non-depressed mothers. Nurses are ideally placed to observe interactions between a mother and child. Does the mother ever play with, or read to, her child? How does the child gain her attention? How does the mother respond to the child's demands? Is the mother irritable and volatile? Is there enjoyable cuddling?

The quality of the mother–child relationship before the onset of depression is an important factor in determining the effects of the depression on the child. Women who have had long-standing difficulties relating to the child show greater breakdown of reciprocal behaviour when under stress; while mothers who are normally competent are not so severely affected in their continuity of care. It appears, therefore, that the preceding personality characteristics of the mother are more important than the episode of depression itself (Mills *et al.*, 1985). Nurses should be aware of these contributory factors in depression and not blame the mother or expect her to 'pull herself together'. She will require support and understanding to progress in her relationship with her child. If maternal depression does have long-lasting effects on the child's cognitive and emotional development, this will be through the altered family relations and persistent disruption of parenting (Puckering, 1989). Maternal depression is often at the root of children's emotional and behavioural problems and nurses in hospital and in the community need to be aware of this possibility and help mothers gain the support they need from the full range of local services.

Disadvantage and social stress

Children from lower social classes tend to do less well at school and have more behaviour problems, but why this is so is not easy to determine. Lower social class often means increased environmental stress in the form of poverty, poor housing conditions, and poor health care and nutrition. The issue here is whether the children's problems and poor intellectual attainment are a result of these adverse conditions, or whether they are determined more by the quality of parenting. A statistical correlation between lower social class and children's increased behaviour problems provides no information on the causal relationship between the two factors; it is important not to jump to conclusions.

In the 1960s and early 1970s, many researchers believed that the reasons for such children's academic failure was due to the lack of cognitive stimulation, the poor level of language between parents and children, and the lack of educational encouragement. This came to represent a 'deficit' model. Attempts to help the children to compensate were made by providing stimulating pre-school experiences in order to enhance language and cognitive development before entry to school.

While the results of these large studies were initially dramatic, the effects seemed to disappear after the children had been at school a few years. Researchers became despondent about the effectiveness of the compensatory pre-school experience. However, they found that as the children moved into the secondary-school age, they did not need as much remedial help as children from the same backgrounds who had not participated in the pre-school programmes. The children also had lower rates of delinquency, and some went on to college. In the long-term follow-up it appeared that the compensatory effect had improved the children's level of self-esteem, their attitude to themselves as learners, and had given them some belief in their own competence (Darlington *et al.*, 1980).

An alternative view is that children from different social and ethnic backgrounds are different rather than deficient in their skills and abilities. Children from other than middle-class social and cultural backgrounds often do less well at school. They may be labelled by teachers, who may expect less of them and may not provide the incentives and opportunities to achieve.

Many children brought up in disadvantaged homes, however, appear to overcome or avoid the consequences of their backgrounds. Longitudinal research that examines children's functioning over several years is needed to elucidate the links between home background and their later social, emotional, and educational problems.

Although general effects have been detected, this does not provide us with clues as to how the social differences cause the effects. It is important for research to move away from the emphasis on social condition in the aetiology of children's problems and to move towards the impact of social conditions on the quality and nature of family life and relationships. We need to question how the effects of social and ethnic background are mediated through the parents' attitudes and behaviour. A parent who has a strong sense of self-esteem, confidence, and identity is likely to enhance the child's view of him or herself and provide a positive attitude towards coping with the problems and stresses of the wider world. Parents who present a model of coping well despite adverse surroundings and experiences help their children to cope more effectively. We must always remember that a large proportion of children from socio-economically stressed families have no social, emotional and educational problems.

Family breakdown

The rate of marital breakdown and divorce has increased sharply during the past 20 years. Because of this, children are experiencing a range of different family structures: they may have two parents early in childhood, then only have a single parent for a while, experiencing a series of transient relationships while the parent is involved with a number of temporary partners. The children may then face the situation of a step-parent joining the family, perhaps with children of their own. If the second marriage does not work out, the whole process may be repeated.

In Britain, it is expected that one in three marriages will break down, and at least one in five children will have experienced divorce by the time they are 16 years old (Donovan, 1984). Between one and two per cent of marriages end each year (Richards, 1988).

The process of family breakdown and divorce can be long and stressful; children may be exposed to distress and conflict for several years before and after the marriage dissolves. It is a period of crisis and uncertainty for all family members, and how it is handled is critical for the child's emotional development (Hetherington, 1989).

Not all separation and divorce is vitriolic. Some parents manage it with sensitivity and consideration for each other and the children. If parents are able to look at the needs of their children and to minimize the effects on them, then the experience need not be so traumatic. Nurses themselves may have experienced the divorce of their own parents or close relatives so it is important for them to develop a realistic rather than a personal perspective about it.

Children who are better able to cope with family breakup have the following positive factors to help alleviate the stress:

- a continuing and stable relationship with both parents;
- a warm and caring relationship with the custodial parent;
- a close relationship with the non-custodial parent;
- good friendships outside the home;
- other sources of emotional support, including grandparents, teachers, and neighbours;
- parents who are psychologically stable. (Wallerstein and Kelly, 1980)

The effects of family breakdown

The emotional climate at home before separation occurs can have a great effect on children's emotional and behavioural state. Living in a home with fighting, angry parents distresses children, who will become involved in the arguments, form alliances, or be used as pawns (Rutter, 1981). Their parents may be moody and unpredictable, or they may suddenly indulge the children with treats in order to gain allegiance, or to alleviate their guilt. Such inconsistencies in the child's world will disrupt normal behavioural and emotional development.

The parents' ability to mediate the effects of the divorce on their children is based on the marital relationship before the divorce. Parents who show greater agreement about child-rearing values and practices also show much less marital disruption, and produce far less disturbance in their children after the divorce (Block *et al.*, 1988). Parents who have vitriolic disputes, often about the custody of the children, cause marked emotional disturbance. Outcome research has given rise to concerns about the ordering of joint custody orders when the parents are continuing to fight. The adverse effects on children's emotional and behavioural states indicate that joint custody and frequent visitation of the other parent is not helpful (Johnston *et al.*, 1989).

Change in living standards

One major effect of divorce is the lowering of living standards for the child and remaining parent. Many women who leave their husbands, taking the children with them, have to go to a women's refuge or stay with friends or relatives. These women and children may then become difficult to link into the community health services because of their transient life style. Some families have to sell their house in order to settle the divorce demands. Or women who may not have worked during their marriage suddenly find themselves trying to find work without qualifications or experience.

Emotional reactions of the custodial parent

Another major effect is that a parent who has been through the trauma of a divorce is often left with immense feelings of anger, depression, failure and anxiety. Because they are coming to terms with these feelings and the divorce, they may have little time to pay attention to their children's emotional needs. Mood swings and inconsistency are common reactions. The parent may also be having difficulty managing the children alone without support. Community health practitioners may need to support a parent through this emotional turmoil in order to maintain care of the children.

The age factor

The age of the child at the time of family breakup is also important. Young children may show behavioural problems like bedwetting and clinging, or regression to more immature behaviour. They may show greater attention-seeking and demands for closeness, but also fewer positive responses such as hugging and smiling, and more negative responses of crying or scowling. Such behaviours can persist for two years after the divorce. These children remain qualitatively different from those of non-divorced parents by having greater social difficulties, greater impulsivity, and attention problems (Hetherington, 1989).

Older school-age children may show anger and aggression towards their parents, and more tearfulness and fearfulness. Adolescents may show depression as an overt response, and also anger, blaming the parent who has left. Some adolescents become precocious in their sexual relationships, and as a result there is a raised incidence of teenage pregnancy and illegitimate births.

Parents may not understand these emotional and behavioural changes in their children and the community health practitioner can take a preventative role in helping parents recognize these effects, and also enable children to talk about their feelings.

The child's age will also determine his or her level of understanding of what has happened. Young children seem to suffer more from marital breakup, which may be due to not understanding what is happening. Parents often don't explain clearly to young children, giving simplistic explanations that don't answer the child's real concerns. Very young children think in a concrete way about relationships: if their parents are living together in the same house, then they are understood to be part of the family. If one parent moves out, however, the child finds it hard to understand that he or she is still a parent. The child may suffer from a sense of bereavement and abandonment, or feel the absent parent no longer loves them, or is angry with them.

In some divorces there is no contact with the non-custodial parent and the child suffers a severe loss of a loved one. Children will also blame themselves for the breakup. Unless this is understood and corrected, the child will continue to feel guilty and anxious about the loss.

Case study

Sarah (aged eight years) had diabetes and had repeated hospitalizations for instability of her blood sugar. Her parents had divorced a
year previously. She told the nurse one night that she thought her
daddy did not love her because of her illness and had left home
because he didn't like her injections.

Children also tend to experience conflicts of loyalty between the
parents, and may feel they have to choose between them. They may
strive and wish continually for a reconciliation, and have great
difficulties accepting that their parents are forming relationships with
other people. The 'good news' of a re-marriage and the prospect of a
step-parent forever kills their hopes of their parents re-uniting and
may lead to an exacerbation of behavioural problems. They may also
fear they could be thrown out or abandoned. The stress and anxiety
that some children experience may result in psychosomatic symptoms.
Occasionally a child's illness will be the reason for the natural parents
to join together in their concern. The nurse should be aware of the
emotional stresses being experienced by children as these can affect
their physical state and health.

Gender

Boys seem to be much more affected by the long-term effects of
divorce than girls (Hetherington, 1989). Because the mother tends to
have custody of the child, boys may lose their fathers at a time when
they need a male authority figure with whom to identify. Girls,
however, also may suffer difficulties in making heterosexual relationships later if no father figure is present (Wallerstein and Kelly, 1980).

Longitudinal studies of the effect of divorce have followed up groups
of children 10 and 15 years post-divorce. They found that many of the
children were still having difficulties working out their own relationships
with the opposite sex, and were intensely frightened about repeating
their parents' unhappy marriage, and continued to identify as 'a child
of divorce' (Wallerstein, 1991).

Case study

Simon's parents had divorced when he was six-years-old after an
acrimonious and prolonged settlement. Simon's father had not
visited him in the ensuing four years, but erratically sent cards and

money to him at birthdays and Christmas. His mother refused to talk about his father to him and he was becoming more anxious and upset about his father's absence as the years progressed. He had started stealing money and showed aggressive and disruptive behaviour at home and school. On the ward he was uncooperative with staff and made up a story that his father would come and 'sort out' the nurses if they made him take his medicine. His behaviour improved once he was encouraged to talk about his father and his mother brought in some photos to show Simon.

Parenting breakdown

When normal parenting patterns and responsibilities break down, the child is exposed to the risk of abuse. This can take many forms – physical, psychological, or sexual – and the abuse may be active or passive.

Table 1.1 *A two-way classification of abuse with examples of major forms (Stratton, 1988)*

	Physical abuse	Psychological abuse	Sexual abuse
Active abuse	Non-accidental injury Poisoning	Emotional abuse Denigration	Incest Rape
Passive abuse	Failure to thrive Poor health care	Neglect Lack of affection	Failure to protect

Psychological abuse and non-accidental injury

Many parents use physical punishment as a discipline and control measure, although this is now being questioned by certain parent pressure groups. When physical punishment is used in extreme measures, the child is considered to be physically abused. Parents who are stretched beyond endurance because of a crying baby can sometimes understand the feelings of rage and desperation that cause some parents to hurt their children.

Child abuse is said to occur when a parent has intentionally hurt their child; however, it is difficult to draw the line between smacking a child hard because they have been naughty, and real abuse. The more extreme forms of abuse are clear – broken limbs, burns, or bruising –

and nurses are now alerted to these signs when treating young children in casualty departments or GPs' surgeries. Parents' claims that the child 'fell downstairs' or 'had an accident' are matched against the child's injuries and the history of previous incidents.

Case study

Tina, aged three years, had a six-month history of doctor's appointments with a dislocated shoulder, a black eye from a fall, and three stitches in a forehead cut. Her health visitor was concerned on visiting the home when she saw bruises on Tina's upper arms and Tina seemed unduly quiet and withdrawn. A new boyfriend of the mother's had moved to the house nine months previously.

The reported incidence of child abuse has been on the increase since the mid-1970s. The gap between the number of reported cases and the number of actual cases is probably narrowing due to an increase in the public's and the professionals' awareness (Creighton, 1988). When looking at incidence figures it is important to consider the growth in general awareness of the community and the extent of investigation of reports; an increase in reporting will include more false interpretations of real accidents, and some malicious allegations.

Difficulties arise in the diagnosis of abuse if the injury to the child was unintentional but was caused by parental neglect, for example a child who was hit by a car when left to play unsupervised. Emotional abuse is even harder to detect and to prove. At present no clear guidelines exist for helping such children. The emotional damage inflicted can be more far-reaching than in physical abuse (Azar *et al.*, 1988). Adults who emotionally abuse their children may be:

- Rejecting (the adult refuses to acknowledge the child's worth).
- Isolating (the child is cut off from normal social experiences, is prevented from forming friendships, or made to feel they are alone in the world).
- Terrorizing (the adult verbally assaults, bullies, and frightens the child repeatedly).
- Ignoring (the adult deprives the child of cognitive and social stimulation, and inhibits their intellectual and emotional growth).
- Corrupting (the child is encouraged and taught to participate in antisocial and deviant behaviour).

Parents who abuse their children fall into no particular category. Abuse occurs across all social classes, ethnic groups, and ages. Although it has been possible through retrospective reports of abusing parents to identify predisposing factors to abuse, there are no clear causal factors, and so it is not yet possible to predict accurately which parents will abuse their children (Roberts, 1988).

Research has identified abusive parents as being impulsive, aggressive, and violent people who have themselves experienced abuse as children, and so repeat their own experiences (Kaufman and Zigler, 1987). Some adults who experienced physical or emotional abuse as children are unable to form good, stable relationships. Abuse is often linked to the adult's poor relationships with their own parents in childhood, and also with sexual frustration within the marriage or partnership. If overwhelmed by social, emotional, and environmental stresses they may take it out on their children. Neglect and abuse often increase with economic tension.

The importance of these associations is that they may help to predict which parents are likely to abuse their children, and so lead to preventative intervention. They also help to indicate which families will benefit from treatment once the abuse has occurred. Decisions about the most appropriate type of intervention and the safe placement of the child may be critical. Unfortunately, preventative strategies have had little effect to date (Browne *et al.*, 1988).

Activity

Find out from one health clinic or GP practice the number of children who are on the child protection register.

Child sexual abuse

Child sexual abuse has received wide publicity in recent years. It is defined as 'the involvement of dependent, developmentally immature children and adolescents in sexual activities they do not truly comprehend, to which they are unable to give informed consent and that violate the social taboos of family roles' (Beezley-Mrazek and Kempe, 1981).

In sexual abuse there is sexual activity between the adult and the child, which is initiated by the adult for his or her own satisfaction. It occurs with children of all ages, and often with young children and babies. About 85 per cent of sexually abused children have been abused by someone they know, often a family member. The child, wishing to please the parent or family friend, becomes confused by the blurring of roles and may feel guilt, shame, or fear, or believe they are in some way responsible.

Recent reports indicate that as many as one in ten of the population in Britain may have experienced some form of sexual abuse as children

(Baker and Duncan, 1985). Patterns of abuse can be repeated through generations, and the experience of one or both parents having been sexually abused as children is the single most common factor in the development of sexual abuse.

The emotional consequences of sexual abuse depend on the age of the child; whether the abuse was accompanied with physical abuse; whether it was long-standing and whether the abuse started gradually or abruptly. How the child's feelings are communicated and managed will also have an effect. Some young children become withdrawn and watchful, others may show sleep disturbance, aggression, and behaviour problems (Hanks *et al.*, 1988). Sudden changes in behaviour or personality may occur, with anxiety, fear, or regression to babyish behaviour. Sudden changes in achievement at school may also be indicative of a traumatic experience. Adolescents may become suicidal or self-mutilating, turn to prostitution and delinquency, or suffer anorexia nervosa and depression (Bentovim *et al.*, 1988).

A pervasive loss of self-esteem is a common characteristic of sexually abused children. This can be shown in mood and behaviour, or through poor self-care. Some children start to neglect their appearance, or exhibit psychosomatic symptoms. A common method of coping is sexualized behaviour, such as seeking sexual contacts, touching teachers or other children intimately, or by displaying inappropriate sexual knowledge through play or drawings.

Due to the breakdown of normal sexual taboos in family life, the child's role becomes distorted and confused. The child may become the provider of adult needs, and may use their 'power' in the family. Or the abused child may be treated as a favourite. The child may cope by taking responsibility for what has happened, carrying a sense of guilt and self-criticism, and may be paralyzed with a fear of retribution if they tell anyone (McFarlane and Waterman, 1986).

The emotional damage that follows sexual abuse lasts through to adult life and may cause the abused adult to then abuse others in turn, or to bury their feelings about the abuse under a sense of guilt and shame, creating problems in emotional and sexual relationships.

The family plays a central role in society, and any analysis of sexual abuse must examine the relationship between the values of society and those of the family. This relationship is complex and not understood: does the family take in the values of the society and transmit them to the children, or does the wider culture reflect the structures and beliefs of its families? The effects of pornography, attitudes to women, and the emphasis on youth all need to be considered.

The taboos on incest and sexual exploitation of children may not be as firmly established as we have supposed. In Western culture the privacy of the family has a high value; people's right to behave as they think fit within their family. The progressive isolation of the family and the loss of contact with the extended family and across generations has had its cost. However, while the isolation of families may be a factor in sexual abuse, extended families who live in close proximity may produce repeated patterns of incest. Although social deprivation is also linked to a higher occurrence of physical and sexual abuse of children, sexual abuse in higher-income families is not unusual.

It appears that the relationship between the parent and child and the parent's own childhood experiences may be important, although it is still not clear whether abuse is purely a matter of sexual drive, or whether it derives from a need to assert power and control, or to retaliate because of feelings of deprivation – or a combination of these. Nurses do encounter sexually abused children and should always keep an open mind to the possibility of this. The recognition and acknowledgement of the high prevalence of child sexual abuse is relatively recent and so nurses need to be alert to the signs and symptoms, and be aware of the procedures for action in their hospital or health authority if they suspect sexual abuse.

Activity
Identify five psychological indicators that a child may have been sexually abused. If you were working in the community, what would you do? Find out the procedures in your local authority and your district health authority for the preliminary stages of liaison about suspected sexual abuse. What should you do if a child mentions to you confidentially that they have been sexually abused?

Bereavement

Many children experience the death of a pet or of a grandparent during early childhood. Some may lose a parent, close friend or sibling, or they may live with a member of the family who is chronically or terminally ill. These experiences will all affect a child's emotional growth, and they will need help to understand what is happening. The nurse should be aware of the impact on the child of serious illness or bereavement in a family in order to support the remaining family members in their grief and help them to talk to the child openly about the events that have made them so upset.

The concept of death

The concept of death is fully developed by around eight years of age. The experience of death in the family, however, enables children who are younger to develop quite advanced notions about death. Children

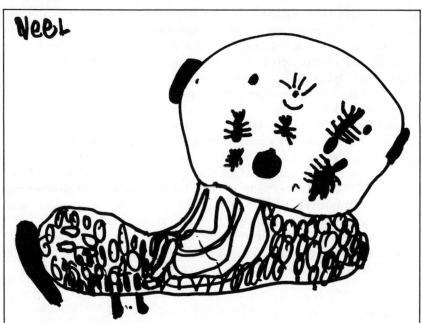

Neel

My cat was in the dog kennel – the dog must have killed it. It got ants all over it and maggots. When animals die – and people – they go underground. It's dirty there and it's dark. I don't want to go there. There are lots of creatures – there are ants and worms and beetles. There are lots of maggots there. When my cat was dead the maggots were all over it – everywhere – and it got ants on its face, nipping it.
Lee (5 years)

of four and five may realize death is a final ending, but may not be too sure that it is irreversible (see Chapter 7).

Pre-school children are often curious about death. They will talk about death without the emotional associations that adults have, and may seem insensitive when others are feeling very sad and upset. Their understanding of death is very concrete and they may ask, for example, whether they can dig up the body to have a look. Or, because they often think death is temporary, they may ask when the dead person is going to come and visit again. They may play games in which they pretend their parents are dead, or that they themselves are dead.

Explaining the cause of death to a child will help him or her to understand what has happened; however, this should match the child's level of understanding of how the body works. It should always be made clear to the child that he or she bears no responsibility for the death. The nurse may be the most well-known person working with

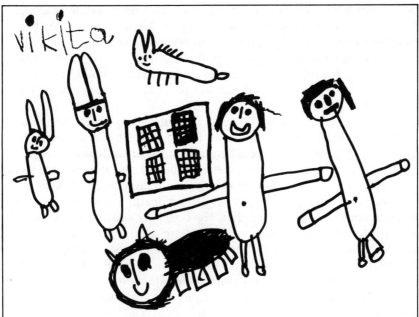

Three people in my family have died – they were very old – you don't die 'til you are very old or very ill. Then you go to heaven – heaven is up in the sky. When your body gets ill and old, it doesn't matter any more – the spirit makes the body sort of float up. When they are up there they look very old. Animals die – there must be cages in heaven to put animals in so they don't escape. They let them out once a day and quickly catch them because they would want to go back down. It rains there but it's okay because there's a roof. It's nice there – you play games.
Nikita (5 years)

the family and so is in a position to alert remaining family members to the needs of the child for age-appropriate information.

Death and religion

Children often ask what happens to people after they die, which can place some parents in a difficult position. The use of religious concepts to explain death is very much the family's decision; parents may tell the child that the dead person 'has gone to heaven', or 'to live with Jesus' or 'Allah'. The adults may not in fact believe this, but use such ideas to stop the child asking awkward questions they do not know how to answer. However, because young children may understand this explanation in a very concrete way, they may ask, for example, why they cannot go to live with Jesus or Allah as well, which can compound the stress that other members of the family are feeling.

School-age children may detect their parents' uncertainty, which can engender more rather than less worry as the child senses that something very important and unmentionable has occurred, which is frightening. Adults should try to express their own understanding of death to the child, and not be concerned about exposing their lack of understanding or confusion. Nurses can facilitate this and help family members to explore their beliefs, uncertainty or confusion.

All religions have their own views on death, and nurses need to be knowledgeable about different beliefs. Sometimes there are very clear guidelines on how a family grieves after a death, following prescribed patterns laid down by the religion. The hospital chaplain should be able to provide information on comparative religions. But nurses should also be aware of the range of beliefs that a family has. Christians have different degrees of belief and so do Muslims, Hindus and other religions. Asking parents and children about their views will help to prevent inappropriate responses from nurses that are based on religious stereotypes.

Exercise

Consider what you might say to a four-year-old child whose dog has just been put down by the vet due to a variety of ailments of old age. How would you explain what had happened? Think about the choice of the phrase 'put to sleep' and what this could mean to the child. What would you say if the child asked if the dog had gone to heaven? Consider the influence of your own religious beliefs on your answer.

The death of a parent

When a child suffers the death of a parent, it may be difficult to disentangle the effect of that loss on the child from the effect of the loss on the remaining parent. The parent's preoccupation with their own feelings may mean the child suffers a double loss: not only the death of one parent, but the lack of attention from the other. Because the bereaved parent has to cope with his or her own grief, there is bound to be a change in their behaviour towards the child (Siegel *et al.*, 1990). For example, the parent may be irritable, depressed, moody, and inconsistent; they may make sudden emotional demands on the child for comfort, or for particularly good and compliant behaviour.

Children show a wide range of problems following the loss of a parent, including high levels of anxiety, separation problems, clinging, excessive crying, aggression, sleeping, eating, and toileting problems. Some children continue to show problems long after the bereavement period, including poor school performance, minor depression and withdrawn behaviour. It is not unusual, however, for some children not to show any grief reactions to a parent's death. This may be due to a denial of the event and the child's inability to come to terms with the immense loss (McCown, 1988).

One prospective study compared a randomly selected group of children aged two to eleven years, 1 and 13 months after the death of a parent. At 1 month there were signs of depressive mood change in over three-quarters of the bereaved children compared with one-third of the non-bereaved controls. By 13 months the reactions in the bereaved group were much less and depressive symptoms were rare, although disinterest in school persisted in some adolescents. These results demonstrate that the immediate consequence of bereavement for children may be severe but of relatively short duration (Van Eerdewegh *et al.*, 1982).

When the death of the parent can be anticipated, preparatory work can be done with the children and the parents. Siegel *et al.* (1990) describe a programme of preventive work with parents dying of cancer that commences six months before the anticipated death. The aim is to support the parents in coping with their own grief, and to enhance their ability to meet their children's heightened need for emotional and physical support. It also provides parents with information about their children's reactions, and how best to talk about the illness while maintaining as much stability and predictability in the children's environment as possible. The work continues with the family for four months after the death of the parent. A number of difficulties with implementing such a programme have been identified, for example, difficulties in estimating the parent's survival time and the problem of engaging families in crisis, and no evaluative data is available yet (Christ *et al.*, 1991). This type of preventative work could be a valuable extension of the role of community health practitioners working with families of terminally ill adults.

The death of a sibling

When children lose a sibling, they may experience a very complex mixture of feelings: they may feel lonely, but also glad they now have their parents all to themselves; young children may feel guilty they caused the death in some way; and some children worry they may catch the same illness or disorder as their sibling and also die.

Case study

Kayleigh (aged 4 years) had a baby sister, Sally, who had died at eight days of age after having been home for three days. This event had been traumatic for the family, but six months later Kayleigh started to talk excessively about Sally and pretend that one of her dolls was Sally. She told her parents, 'If you have another baby, I'll look after it and she'll be alright'. Her distress and concerns had taken a long time to emerge and created a situation where the parents had to go over the death all over again with Kayleigh to help her remember and understand it.

Some of the child's behavioural problems may in fact be a reflection of the parents' mourning process. They can become preoccupied with the dead child and unwittingly deprive the living child of attention, care, and love; or they may subconsciously blame the living child for still being alive; or they may idealize the dead child to the detriment of its sibling. Sometimes, fearing another loss, parents become overprotective of the living child and do not allow them to become independent (Rosen, 1986). The community health practitioner should be alert to the effects on the remaining children after the death of a sibling and intermittent visiting over a long period after the death may be necessary to identify continuing difficulties.

Mourning

Children need help to understand death and grief. They need to be allowed to mourn the lost person, and not to be denied the opportunity to cry or to talk about their feelings, or their experiences with and memories of the dead person.

Some adults feel children should be protected from death and not be allowed to see adults mourning. However, secrecy around these issues will make children feel worried and suspicious, or even guilty about what has happened. The adults should be able to cry and share their feelings of sadness with the child – as long as this does not overwhelm or frighten the child (McCown, 1988).

In one study, six family-therapy sessions were offered to bereaved children and the remaining parent. The aim of the session was to promote a normal mourning process in the children and the parent, and to improve communication between them, especially about the death. The group of families that received treatment were compared to a control group one year and two years after the bereavement. After the first year follow-up, the treatment-group children were significantly less likely to be restless, bite their nails, or to have depressed parents.

The mothers from the treatment group were less likely to have sought help from professional agencies. By the second year, the treatment group showed significantly fewer health-related problems in the surviving parents. A favourable outcome was associated with the child having cried and talked about the dead parent in the month following the death. Parents who showed emotional problems after the death tended to inhibit the child talking (Black and Urbanowitz, 1987).

It appears to be important to assess the well-being of the surviving parents, and to intervene when necessary. There may be a mediating influence of parental mental health on a child's well-being following bereavement, and other life events carrying a potentially severe impact (McFarlane, 1988).

The bereaved child needs order and routine in his or her life, and should be encouraged to continue with normal activities after the death. They also need some time for themselves with caring adults to make it clear how important they still are, and that the disruption to the normal routine has not changed the adults' feelings towards them. Adolescents may need time to consider the implications of the death in terms of their philosophy of life, and also their views of the future. Particularly at this age there may be a heightened sensitivity to death, and a fuller understanding of what death really means and their own mortality (Corr and McNeil, 1986).

Guidelines for nurse intervention

There are three main conclusions to the general findings from research into the effects of bereavement and divorce. First, the impact on the parents must be evaluated in order to assess the impact on the children. It is not clear whether some children are affected because of existing vulnerability factors such as a past history of disturbance or poor family relations, or whether the event is sufficiently distressing in itself. From the nurse's point of view, the type of life event, its social impact on the family, and the personal meaning it has for the child will all be important in determining the type of intervention and help required to prevent problems developing and being maintained.

Secondly, it appears that crying and talking are important in promoting good adjustment, and these need to be encouraged even when a substitute parent joins the family. The process of developing a reconstituted family can prevent healthy adjustment, and the child may be silenced rather than coming to terms with the loss of a parent.

Thirdly, some of the adverse consequences of bereavement can be diminished by help reaching families at the right time; intervention can shorten the period of distress. It may be appropriate for bereavement counselling to be offered as a primary prevention service; however there are questions about whether only families demonstrating abnormal grief reaction should be offered help, or whether all families suffering a bereavement should be screened for difficulties (Goodyer, 1990).

The main practical guidelines for health professionals working with grieving children include the following:

- The child should be told about the death as soon as possible in truthful, clear, and simple terms appropriate to his or her level of understanding.
- The adults should feel free to share their feelings of sadness with the child in a controlled manner.
- The child should be encouraged to discuss, question, and express feelings about the event and experiences surrounding the death.
- A specific pattern of grief should not be imposed on the child.
- The care-taking needs of the child should continue to be met by a warm and loving person.
- The child should be given a choice regarding funeral attendance.
- Time with the child and loved adults should be set aside in the immediate days after the death in order to assure the child of his or her continuing values and importance.
- Other important people in the child's life should be told of the death, for example teachers.
- The child should be encouraged to resume normal activities after the death.
- At each new cognitive, developmental level the child will need to review and reinterpret the loss in the light of new growth and understanding (McCown, 1988).

The Childhood Death Awareness Inventory has been developed to help the health professional to open up communication about death in the family. It moves from direct questioning about the death to explanations that have been given to the child, e.g., 'What has the child been told about the disposal of the body?' Supportive measures that are needed to help the grieving child are then explored (McCown, 1988).

Table 1.2 *Childhood Death Awareness Inventory (from McCown, 1988)*

Family Name _____   Date _____

Address _____

_____

Child's Name _____   Age _____

Name of Deceased _____   Age _____

Relationship to Child _____

Date of Death _____

I. **Child's experience with death**: What experiences has the child had with death?

  A. Pet(s) _____ Date of death _____

    Child's reaction and comments: _____

  B. Distant Relative _____ Date of death _____

    Name _____ Relationship _____

    Child's reaction and comments: _____

  C. Close Relative _____ Date of death _____

    Name _____ Relationship _____

    Child's reaction and comments: _____

  D. Friends _____ Date of death _____

    Name _____ Relationship _____

    Child's reaction and comments: _____

  E. Community (teacher, pastor, schoolmates)

    Name _____ Date of death _____

    Relationship _____

    Child's reaction and comments: _____

II. **Rituals of death**

  A. Has the child seen a dead person?   Yes _____ No _____

  B. Has the child seen a dead animal?   Yes _____ No _____

  C. Has the child attended a funeral or memorial service?   Yes _____ No _____

  D. Has the child visited a cemetery?   Yes _____ No _____

III. **Beliefs about death**

  A. What beliefs about death are held by the child? _____

  B. What beliefs about death are held by the family? _____

  C. Is the child familiar with the church (synagogue) building?   Yes _____ No _____

IV. **Explanation of death**

  A. What has the child been told about the death? _____

  B. What has the child been told about the disposal of the body? _____

  C. What has the child been told about the final services (funeral, memorial service)? _____

V. **Expected reaction**

  A. How do you expect (child) to respond to the loss? _____

  B. What adjustments will be difficult for the child? _____

VI. **Supportive measures**

  A. What actions will comfort your child? _____

Table 1.2 *Continued*

B. Who are the people who can help your child? Have you notified them of
    the death? _____

C. What literature have you read about death and grief? _____

D. What questions do you have about your child and death? _____

Long-term follow-up of bereaved families can be very meaningful, and help to strengthen the supportive relationship with them. The child's behaviour can be reviewed with the family, and any children with prolonged or multiple problems can be identified for referral for specialist help in order to avoid long-term emotional disturbances.

Summary

This chapter links the reader's understanding of the growing and changing child with the most important experience of the child's life – the family. The child's emotional, social, and intellectual growth is determined by experiences within the family. Parents often determine the child's exposure and adjustment to religious, cultural and social expectations so, in nursing the children of a multicultural society, with its many styles and variations of family life, nurses need to be conscious of the different experiences that children face, and should not use a personal experience of family life as a standard for all others. Children's behaviour and emotional state reflects their family upbringing, and nurses meet a number of children who have been damaged by that experience.

Issues around attachment and bonding have had a significant effect on nursing practice and these concepts have created a framework for understanding the problems encountered in families when there is a breakdown in the parenting role resulting in abuse. Children also face a range of other difficulties, i.e. parental divorce, or bereavement, that create significant stresses resulting in behavioural and emotional problems. These stresses are often in addition to the problems encountered by acute or chronic illness, and nurses should consider the effect of these on the child during the period of nursing care. The implications for the management and psychological support of the child and family are considerable.

Further reading

Browne, K., Davies, C., and Stratton, P. (1988). *Early Prediction and Prevention of Child Abuse*. Chichester, John Wiley.
Provides a thoughtful look at the community health-care issues in child-abuse work. The problems of screening, predicting, preventing, and treating child abuse are presented in a way that makes the reader aware of the complexity of the issues involved, and that there are no simple answers.

Goodyer, I. M. (1990). Family relationships, life events and childhood psychopathology. *J. of Child Psychology and Psychiatry, (31),* 161–92.
Presents a very coherent and comprehensive account of research related to the effect of family life and life events on the child's emotional, behavioural and cognitive development.

Rutter, M. (1985). Family and school influences on behavioural development. *J. of Child Psychology and Psychiatry, (26),* 349–69.
An analysis of findings of research related to the environmental effects on children's behavioural development. Discusses possible mechanisms and processes by which these effects can be understood, and identifies the areas needed for further research.

Wallerstein, J. S. (1991). The long term effects of divorce on children: a review. *J. of the American Academy of Child and Adolescent Psychiatry, (30),* 349–60.
A comprehensive review of all American research studies on the effects of divorce. Provides a readable overview, plus a brief outline of each of the major research initiatives.

2 *Primary health care of children in the community*

Introduction

The role of the nurse is changing in line with the current trends in primary health care. Nurse education now acknowledges the importance of community and family care, and stresses the need to understand the whole person – physically, intellectually, emotionally, and socially.

In order to promote good health care of children, nurses need to work with families to facililtate the skills, time, and concern of the parents. Helping the parents to take more responsibility and to increase their awareness of how to bring up healthy children are vital aspects of the community health professional's job.

Do we have to wait for a child to be abused before help can be offered to parents? Does the family of a disabled or mentally handicapped child have to break up before support and counselling are offered? Does a child have to be admitted to hospital for prolonged periods because the family does not have the support needed to look after their chronically ill child? Help is often required *before* the crisis occurs, and awareness of the factors contributing to the breakdown of family support for children is very important.

Community health care

An historical emphasis on acute care rather than preventative work has diverted attention away from the effects of environmental and social factors on health. We know, however, that social class, gender, race and geography are all determinants of the level of health and health care in Britain today. In fact, the effects of medical services are secondary to social and economic influences such as income, housing, working conditions, education, unemployment, nutrition, and the quality of the environment and local amenities.

Different racial groups also have different needs. For example, the incidence of certain illnesses is higher in particular groups, and only certain groups are susceptible to particular illnesses. Dietary patterns and reactions to drugs also vary between ethnic groups (Henderson

50

and Primeaux, 1981). The health care offered may be unacceptable for religious or cultural reasons, for example a mother may be reluctant to see a male doctor. Past experiences of prejudice and discrimination can also affect parents' expectations of the health service, as well as their co-operation and compliance.

We know that families in the lower socio-economic groups have more health problems than families in higher socio-economic groups, and that they require a disproportionate amount of health service resources. It also appears that the families and children most in need of health services are least likely to receive or use them and, conversely, those who least need services are most likely to receive them. Ethnic minority communities in particular are likely to be affected by these factors, which may be exacerbated by direct or indirect discrimination. The Children Act (HMSO, 1989) now specifies clearly that the health service offered to the child and family should be appropriate to the child's race, culture, religion and language, with staff working in partnership with parents.

Understanding the context of children's health problems is crucial in providing effective prevention, remediation or treatment. Health and sickness are affected by the child's life-style, family, where they live, past experiences, and personality. Children from families living in poor housing conditions, with low income, or unemployment, and a low level of parental education, have an increased risk of poor health, along with learning difficulties, and behavioural and emotional problems. Children from homeless families and those who live in overcrowded conditions, with poor sanitation, inadequate cooking facilities, and inadequate play areas are especially susceptible to poor health. The families also may not be registered with the local health services and so miss out on basic health care (Ashton and Seymour, 1988).

Primary health care: the aims

Primary health care today depends on community participation and collaboration between agencies. In aiming to eliminate inequalities in health care, the World Health Organization (WHO) has identified three main objectives (WHO Europe 1981, 1985):

➤ To promote healthy life-styles

By developing individual awareness of health risks and changes in behaviour needed to improve health, the emphasis is placed on improving social and economic conditions that affect the life-styles of families, including job opportunities, working and living conditions and social networks. The aim is also to help the public to make healthy choices by providing information and educating families about health issues, and through legislative and regulatory controls such as dietary advice and the labelling of food contents.

➤ To prevent preventable conditions

Mothers and children require adequate primary health care through perinatal, maternal, infant and child care, and family planning and genetic counselling. The emphasis is on the early detection of defects and risk factors. All children should be covered by an appropriate immunization programme. An awareness of safety will reduce accidents inside and outside the home. Nutritional education for parents and children will discourage bad eating habits and, of course, safe water and sanitation are essential.

➤ To provide rehabilitation and health services

All families should have access to community-based primary health care. This should emphasize preventative medicine, health promotion, self-help, and self-care. The high-risk groups — the mentally handicapped, mentally ill, disabled, and elderly — require special services, and there should be early diagnosis and intervention to prevent chronic and degenerative disease.

There is currently a move away from a predominantly medical view of health services towards a holistic view of health in the community by encouraging:

- an increase in self-care;
- the integration of medical care with education, recreation, environmental improvements, and social welfare;
- the integration of good health promotion with preventative medicine, treatment, and rehabilitation;
- meeting the needs of under-served groups;
- increasing community participation.

Health promotion is a key element. It requires a broad-based approach that will enable parents to increase their control over and improve their own and their children's health. Community health practitioners need to be aware of strategies and ways of working that will facilitate these changes. Primary medical care should provide an accessible prevention and treatment service and, where possible, mobilize public participation and inter-agency working, involving a range of people other than health workers to promote health.

Community nursing: the aims

The health professional working in the community performs a wide range of roles while delivering a primary health care service. The following aims of community nursing will be discussed from a primarily psychological point of view.

1. To provide a good standard of 'primary' health care to all families in the community.
2. To participate in the identification and prevention of behavioural, emotional, developmental and health problems.
3. To assess social, emotional, and psychological factors contributing to health problems in children.
4. To facilitate self-help and self-care for parents and their children.
5. To understand and link with different agencies within the community.

1. *Good health care for all*

Primary health care should meet the social, cultural and ethnic needs and expectations of the parents. Being sensitive to the family's child-rearing views and relationship and dietary patterns, is essential. Cultural and social stereotypes are often very inaccurate descriptions of the individual differences that exist in families. Health professionals need to be aware of personal biases about the families they prefer or prefer not to visit, and that their attitudes and ideas may stem from their own cultural and social class.

Case study

When one health visitor recorded the time spent on visits to each family she found to her surprise that she spent considerably longer with mothers that she enjoyed talking to than with mothers who were less communicative. She also became aware that the tension she felt when due to visit some difficult families was relieved when she found that they were not in. She admitted that she often hoped they would be out.

Eye contact, expressions, head and body movements, physical distance, and touch can all be misunderstood. Tone of voice, loudness, speed and pitch can be misinterpreted, and lead to strong feelings.

Because of this, interpreters, both in clinics and on home visits, are often necessary. It is the nurse's responsibility to arrange this. The nurse should get to know the interpreter so that the aims of the discussion are understood; to ensure that the interpreter is fluent in both languages; to make the interpreter aware that some topics may be distressing or embarrassing; and to emphasize that the interpreter should translate exactly what is said.

Many parents cannot read or write English. Letters for appointments should take account of poor literacy and different languages – if parents do not attend appointments, it may be because they cannot read or understand the letter that has been sent. Parents are usually embarrassed about this, and it is therefore inappropriate to ask outright if they can read. A sensitive and supportive, rather than confrontational, approach is more helpful.

2. *Identification and prevention*

The prevention of behavioural, emotional, developmental and health problems in children is an important part of community health care. Primary prevention includes health education within the community while secondary prevention aims to identify the children at risk or who already have problems. Before prevention can take place, however, the problems must be identified.

Identification of problems: screening

Screening procedures are used to identify pre-school children at risk of developmental and health problems in the community, e.g. developmental checklists and hearing and vision tests. Although these are used on community populations in general health surveillance, it is questionable whether screening for psycho-social problems is possible or worthwhile, as it may not be accurate or cost-effective.

The sensitivity and specificity of any screening instrument, whether it is a checklist or a specific test, is critical for its predictive value. With any screening instrument it is possible to have false positives (children identified as having problems when they have not) and false negatives (children who have problems but who are not identified). In the first case, the children are labelled inappropriately; and in the second, children who require help may not receive it. Deciding the cut-off point to identify a child at risk of developmental or language problems is difficult as there are wide variations in the normal range of ability. If the sensitivity of the screening instrument is low, the majority of true positives will not be identified: if the specificity is low, then the majority of true negatives will not be identified.

Instead of screening the entire community, it can be more cost-effective to select children for preventative intervention on the basis of their own or their family's characteristics, for example, chronic medical illness, frequent hospitalization, divorcing parents, or a death in the family. However, as only a minority of these children will develop behavioural or emotional problems, there is still the risk of offering preventative work to families who do not need it.

Psychological screening assessments

Developmental screening identifies children at risk of developmental and language problems so that appropriate services can be directed to the families. Simple developmental tests like the Denver are used by health visitors in homes and clinics, but there is wide variation in policy on who should carry out developmental screening and how intensively (DHSS, 1986). Health visitors and primary health care teams can be instrumental in obtaining services for children with suspected developmental difficulties by referring on to specialists for further assessment and intervention. For example, nursery provision can be recommended to provide stimulation for the child and relief for stressed parents, or admission is arranged to special opportunity groups for children with special needs.

Screening for early behaviour problems can be carried out by using one of the wide range of parent-completed checklists, for example the *Behaviour Screening Questionnaire*, suitable for three-year-olds (Richman and Graham, 1971); the *Children's Behaviour Checklists*, for children 2–4 and 4–7 years (Achenbach and Edelbrock, 1983); the *Behaviour Checklist*, suitable for three-year-olds (Richman, 1977); the *Pre-School Behavioural Questionnaire* (Behar and Stringfield, 1974); and finally, the *Behaviour Checklist*, for children nine months to two years of age (Hewett, 1990). These checklists can identify pre-school children exhibiting behaviour difficulties and who therefore may be at risk of later behavioural problems.

The number of problems identified by parents far exceeds the available resources for treatment, so the value of providing routine screening for behaviour problems is questionable. However, knowledge about the extent of behaviour problems in children in the community is still necessary for health professionals to plan resources and create intervention programmes. Thus, the identification of behavioural and emotional problems in defined high-risk groups using multiple measures may be a better use of professional time: resources can then be targeted more precisely, and evaluation of the intervention developed.

Table 2.1 *Example of a multiple criteria screen for mother and toddler for emotional and behavioural problems (Nicol et al., 1987)*

Nicol *et al.* (1987) have described the development of a multiple criteria screen for mother and toddler problems which used three measures:

a) the *General Health Questionnaire* (Goldberg, 1988) to select a group of mothers at risk for mental health problems
b) the *Behaviour Checklist* (Richman, 1977) to identify young children with behaviour problems
c) a health visitors' questionnaire to collect data from existing health visitors' information on the families.

The criterion of a 'case' was a level of mother or toddler disorder that merited active treatment at primary care level. The results of the screening instruments were rated against a psychiatrist's diagnosis of the severity of mother and toddler disorder from an interview. The sensitivity of the screen was found to be very high (94.9%) although the specificity was lower (61.88%) i.e. it was too inclusive and so identified children without problems.

true positives	false positives
223.88	205.77
true negatives	false negatives
333.97	12.04

Screening to identify children at risk of abuse is becoming an important indicator of community psychological health. A number of risk factors have been identified in families who have abused their children, and attempts have been made to predict from these which families in the general population are most at risk. Standard screening procedures should be used with caution because of cultural and social differences e.g. the level of physical punishment used by parents varies widely between different communities.

Browne and Saqi (1988a) describe a well-designed, retrospective study that was carried out with health visitors in 1983 by Browne and Stevenson to complete a 13-item risk-factors checklist on all children under five years who had been identified as suffering physical abuse and neglect. Information was collected on 62 families. The health visitor then selected 62 control non-abusing families from the same district who matched the abusing families in socio-demographic characteristics, and so had a matched control sample of 124 families (Table 2.2).

The risk factors in Table 2.2 are listed in order of relative importance. The most predictive factor was the health visitor's perception of whether the parent was indifferent, intolerant, or over-anxious. The final three factors did not reach statistical significance.

Table 2.2 *Risk-factors checklist for abusing families (Browne and Stevenson, 1983)*

1. Parents who are indifferent, intolerant, or over-anxious towards their children.
2. A history of family violence.
3. Socio-economic problems in the family, e.g. unemployment.
4. The child having been premature or of low birth weight.
5. The parent having been abused or neglected as a child.
6. Step-parent or cohabitee present.
7. Single or separated parents.
8. Mother less than 21 years old at the birth of the child.
9. History of mental illness, drug or alcohol addiction in the parents.
10. The baby having been separated from the mother for more than 24 hours post-delivery.
11. Infant mentally or physically handicapped. (No significant difference.)
12. Less than 18 months between the birth of children. (No significant difference.)
13. Infant never breast fed. (No significant difference.)

When completing a checklist like Table 2.2, of course it is not possible to simply add up the number of significant factors present in a family. Some factors are more significant than others; all cannot be given the same importance. Even with the maximum possible performance, a checklist such as this used as a screening instrument is only sensitive to 82% of abusing families and 88% of non-abusing families. This is not clinically acceptable because 18% of abusing families are not being identified, and 12% are being wrongly identified as abusing.

The next stage was to see whether the checklist could be used predictively on a routine basis for primary prevention. One prospective study was carried out completing the checklist on 14,238 births in Surrey between 1984–5. The families were then followed up for five years. The checklist was presented in the form of a bar scale for each risk factor, so the health visitor could indicate the severity of the concern. The midwife completed the scale at the birth of the child, and the health visitor completed it during the first month of life. Two years later, 6.7% of the population were considered 'high-risk', but only 6% of those 'high-risk' families went on to abuse their child, indicating a high number of false positives. There were also changes in risk factors during the first two years of the child's life. The researchers concluded that background influences and stress are not sufficient explanations for child abuse and neglect (Browne and Saqi, 1988a).

Another approach focuses more on the parent–child relationship by observing mothers and infants at home and requesting mothers to fill in a child-behaviour checklist. It was found that abusing mothers have significantly more negative perceptions of their infants than non-abusing mothers. By observing brief separations and reunions of mother and child, it was found that mother–infant interaction in abusing families is less reciprocal and more coercive than in controls (Browne and Saqi, 1987). Abusing families also have a higher proportion of anxiously attached children (70%) compared to controls (26%) (Browne and Saqi, 1988b). This type of research, however, has not yet provided the community health professional with a simple method of predicting accurately which families are likely to abuse their children.

Screening for child abuse is a complex and costly process. In order to eliminate false alarms, one suggestion is that it should involve three stages:

1. All new parents should be screened after the birth for social and demographic characteristics of the child and family. This will identify a target group, but will miss some.
2. Three to six months after the birth, all parents in the target group should be screened on their perceptions of the baby, and which aspects of parenting and family life they find stressful.
3. Nine to twelve months after the birth, the baby's attachment to the main caregiver and the parental sensitivity to the baby's behaviour should be assessed (Browne and Saqi, 1988a).

Prevention

Once the problems have been identified, prevention programmes can be devised. Two types of community prevention programmes have been described: primary prevention aims to reduce the incidence of new cases in a population; secondary prevention aims to reduce the number of existing cases.

Primary prevention

Offord (1987) has reviewed a number of primary prevention programmes aimed at children's behavioural and emotional problems. He sees primary prevention as: building up strengths in the child (for example, increasing the child's competence); reducing the harmful effects of a stressful environment (for example, reducing the stress of divorce); and increasing the health-enhancing aspects of the family or community (for example, programmes that aim to increase social support for families). He further classifies primary prevention programmes into three types:

a) Educational programmes for children of a certain age or developmental level such as *Head Start* in the United States. *The Perry Pre-school Project* in North America provided a pre-school educational programme for economically disadvantaged children of below average intellectual ability and was directed at their educational and social development. The children were assigned randomly to experimental or control groups. When the children were aged 19, follow up revealed better academic achievement for the experimental group compared to the control group, and also some advantages in emotional adjustment, such as fewer arrests by the police. Increased academic success had enabled at risk children to become better socially adjusted (Berreuta-Clement *et al.*, 1984).

b) High-risk programmes for children who are at increased risk of disorder; for example, the *Divorce Adjustment Project* in the USA provided a 12 session psycho-educational programme for children and 12-week support groups for parents. There was a reported increase in self-esteem and positive social behaviour among the children, and improved adjustment to being divorced among the parents (Stolberg and Garrison, 1985).

c) Community-wide programmes which focus on an entire population of children in a specific geographical area or a particular school. Outcome measures are not restricted to individual children, but include community measures such as vandalism rates, number of police calls, and so on.

Unfortunately, there have been no clear or unequivocal positive results from large scale primary prevention studies. Such studies are time consuming, costly and extremely difficult to do because of the low incidence of emotional and behavioural problems in the general population, and sample sizes need to be extremely large to demonstrate important differences that are attributable to intervention.

Secondary prevention

One secondary prevention programme selected families 'at risk' using the multiple screening technique in Table 2.1 and then allocated them to a mother-and-toddler group for ten sessions (Nicol *et al.*, 1987). The mothers also participated in a group session separate from their toddlers. The project compared peer-group support with special-health visiting and family therapy. No comparative evaluative data is yet available, but a follow-up questionnaire confirmed that the mothers had found the groups helpful in understanding their children and their own reactions, and had appreciated the emotional support.

Health professionals should consider the best way of providing preventative services to the community, and try different types of service provision. It is important not to adopt a single or standard method, but to try out different forms of contact with families. Evaluation of those contacts will provide insight into the effectiveness of the service, and whether the target group is being reached.

One primary health care team introduced an appointments system at a well-baby clinic where the mother could see a health visitor individually. The team also tried a six-week postnatal support group for first-time mothers. Results indicated the mothers required less health-visiting time at the clinic, and requested very few house calls (Moulds *et al.*, 1983a, b). A recent initiative is Childline, which has contributed to the primary prevention of child abuse by bringing it to the public's and professionals' attention. However, as only 1.5% of children were referred on for professional help in the first eight months, questions have been raised about its usefulness as a method of bringing abused children into the network of professional help. It is an extensive, but possibly expensive, form of screening and assessment for child abuse and neglect.

3. *Assessment of psychological factors contributing to health problems in children*

When a parent presents his or her child as having a health problem, it is important to understand the multitude of influences that can affect the child's health, and to widen the assessment beyond physical and biological factors. Psychological factors may play an important role: for example, a child may continue to soil him or herself in junior school in order to unite the parents in their concern and divert attention from a marital problem; or a mother may need to have a 'sick' child in order to gain support from local or hospital services because she has nowhere else to turn for consideration of her own needs.

Assessment can use formal instruments for measuring problems, or checklists and semi-structured interviews such as the one in Table 2.3.

4. *Facilitating self-help and self-care*

It will never be possible to support a comprehensive, individually-based health service. The community or groups within the community must take control and responsibility for their own health needs. This can be enhanced by the community health practitioner encouraging community participation in the planning and delivery of health services (Orr, 1985). As well, through the sharing of experiences and coping strategies, skills can be developed and enhanced without recourse to professional intervention. An excellent example of this has been the New Parent Infant Network Model (NEWPIN). NEWPIN was

---

Table 2.3 *Topics for a semi-structured interview*

Community level
- What are the housing, employment, economic, and stress levels in the community?
- How isolated is the family from networks within the community, service agencies, and relatives?
- What cultural, religious, ethnic, and social networks are available within the community?

Family level
- What previous experiences might be affecting the parents' present reactions (including level of education and social, family, and emotional experiences)?
- What is the quality of the home environment, i.e. level of cleanliness and organization?
- Are there any present or past marital and relationship difficulties?
- Do parents have any emotional or mental health difficulties?
- What is the present structure of family relationships, including the extended family?
- How effective are the parents at parenting their child?
- How good is the parent–child relationship?
- What style of child management do the parents use?

Child level
- Does the child show behaviour problems?
- How does the health or behaviour problems affect the child's normal social life at home or in school?
- How does the problem affect the child's self-esteem, confidence, and view of him or herself?
- How does the child's emotional state affect the child's health and behaviour?

---

established in 1982 in a deprived neighbourhood in London. Its aim was to meet the needs for friendship, support, and practical assistance of inner-city families with young children. Volunteers, recruited from the local community, receive a brief training and group supervision and support from a visiting group therapist. The volunteers are paired with client mothers, who have been referred by health visitors, social workers, or GPs because of depression, isolation, or problems in parenting. The volunteers bring mothers to the NEWPIN drop-in centre, where there is a playroom with a playleader, and a sitting-room for the parents. Mothers have reported a growth in self-esteem, self-confidence, and relationships with others, proving that a volunteer organization with only one full-time professional worker is able to influence a large number of families (Pound and Mills, 1985).

Exercise

Identify four goals you would have in establishing a parents' discussion group on young children's behaviour problems in your health centre. Consider three different ways of evaluating the outcome of such a group. (Suggested answers at end of book.)

Self-help groups

Many health visitors see the facilitating of mother-and-toddler groups to discuss problems of general child management as an integral part of their work (Carpenter, 1990). Mothers may be supported to create their own self-help discussion group about life with toddlers; or a parent group may wish to learn more about their own and their children's health. Billingham (1989) identified a group of teenage parents and developed a support group to enhance parenting skills, to provide an opportunity to learn about children, and to increase self-esteem.

Voluntary and support groups

Supporting parents in the contacting of voluntary groups and the myriad groups for children's specific disorders and illnesses is another vital role for the nurse in the community; talking with the group members can be of great benefit.

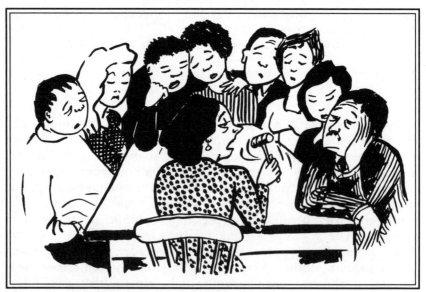

I declare this meeting – of the Support Group of Parents Whose Children Have Sleep Problems – open!

Play groups and family centres

The nurse may need to be a catalyst in mobilizing resources within the community by setting up play groups, family centres, or home-based groups for mutual support. One such group had six to eight members and a leader who was also a mother. They met in each other's home, and came together for larger social events. There was a monthly newsletter, and a library of books bought by fundraising. The results of interviewing the 43 mothers indicated that the groups helped to prevent social isolation and psychosomatic illness as the families gave mutual support and the mothers had friends to whom they could turn (Hiskins, 1981).

There are also groups for parents' problems such as alcoholism, single-parent families, battered wives, and women's support groups. Helping families to link with one of these might offset the development of serious family problems that could, in turn, affect a child adversely. Drop-in centres for women's preventative health care may also have an effect on psychological health (May, 1989).

The community health practitioner should be fully aware of the range of parent-support groups that exist both locally and nationwide. A resource list should be compiled from the library, social services, educational services, from talking with parents, and from books and articles on children's problems. The health professional should understand what these groups offer and how they are organized in order to facilitate a new parent joining and taking advantage of the services being offered.

Ethnic needs

The importance of social support groups is often accentuated in ethnic minority areas. Mothers from different cultural backgrounds, many of whom do not speak English, may live isolated lives, cut off from their friends and relatives. The role of women and the control exerted by the husband needs to be considered cautiously, and to be respected. Here, contacts with community-based ethnic minority workers and organizations can help ease the cultural gap and aid the health professional in understanding and helping isolated mothers gain the support they need. Community support groups based on ethnic needs are important, as well as groups that integrate across cultural groups. In many communities, parents work to educate each other and their children about different cultural patterns, for example by organizing displays of food, stories, customs, and costumes from various countries. For older children, films from different cultures and religions may be shown in schools or in youth centres.

By not focusing only on the clinical needs of the children and families, the health professional's role is to extend the health care contacts by publicizing and disseminating information, reaching as wide a section of the community as possible through parent-support groups; combining efforts with other agencies in the community; and contacting families who otherwise would not contact health services, e.g. traveller families and those who fail to attend child health surveillance (Children Act, 1989).

5. Understanding and linking with the community network of agencies

The nurse is part of a network of primary care services that includes health, social services, and education. Because many decisions involving children and families are multidisciplinary in nature, co-operation and the exchange of information between agencies is vital so that children do not fall between areas of responsibility, and are not overlooked. Often, problems arise which are outside the nurse's area of knowledge or expertise, and it is necessary to obtain additional help. The Children Act (1989) specifies the value of different agencies co-operating, consulting and keeping each other informed. Appropriate packages of services involving different agencies may need to be developed in partnership with the family and child.

Community health services

The provision of service will vary across the country. Community health practitioners should find out what is available in their area.

- General practitioners: some GP surgeries are developing primary care teams with practice nurses, health visitors, and clinical psychologists linked to them (Bowling and Stilwell, 1988).

- Community health clinics: these are used for health care of the under-fives, for weighing babies, providing nutritional advice, health and development checks, and immunizations. A senior clinical medical officer or a community paediatrician may hold clinics there.

- Hospital services: children have access to specialist paediatricians as well as therapy specialities such as physiotherapists, speech and language therapists, occupational therapists, clinical psychologists, child psychiatrists, and dietitians.

- Child guidance units: when a child shows behavioural and emotional problems at home or at school, then referral to a child guidance unit is made. Children of all ages are seen, and a variety of therapeutic interventions is available, including family therapy, behaviour therapy and psychotherapy, depending on the orientation of the clinic. Families may be able to see a child psychiatrist, a psychiatric social worker, an educational or clinical psychologist, or a psychotherapist. Clinics often accept referrals from parents, or from schools, GPs, or health visitors.

- Child development centres: these do not exist all over Britain, and may or may not be linked to the district handicap team. Their purpose is to provide a multidisciplinary assessment and treatment centre for children with physical and developmental handicaps, as well as medical treatment; the provision of aids and resources; advice, counselling, and support to parents and families; and therapy intervention. The professionals involved may include any of the following: community paediatrician, health visitor, social worker, speech and language therapist, clinical or educational psychologist, physiotherapist, occupational therapist, senior clinical medical officer, audiologist, teacher.

Activity
Find the name and address of the Child Development Centre in your area and request information on the range of services offered. How is a child referred to that centre? How effective is liaison with the community health practitioners?

Social services

Children defined as being in need will have a social worker based in the local social services department. Social workers may work in generic teams, or have specialist teams for child and family work or children with special needs. Because local authority areas may not match the health districts, community nurses may have contact with several different social workers working with families in their areas. A child in need is one who is 'unlikely to achieve or maintain, or to have the opportunity of achieving or maintaining, a reasonable standard of health or development without the provision for him of services by the local authority' (HMSO, 1989).

Although social workers have various statutory duties to carry out for the care and protection of children in families, legislation frequently changes as has occurred recently with the Children Act.

The Children Act (1989) has specified that the social services department has two general duties with respect to children in need:

1) to safeguard and promote their welfare;

2) to promote their upbringing by their families provided it is in the child's best interests.

In addition to these are specific duties and powers:

● to identify the extent to which there are children in need in their area;
● to have regard to the different racial groups to which children in their area who are in need belong, when making arrangements for the provision of day care, or to encourage persons to act as local authority foster parents;
● to provide services for children in need living with their own families;
● to provide accommodation for children in need;
● to prevent neglect and abuse by the provision of services;
● to reduce the need, by provision of services, to bring court proceedings.

Community health practitioners need to be aware of the definition of children in need and their own role in defining this. They may be involved in the assessment of the child, identification of need in the area and in liaising with the social services department in providing services. Health professionals now have a duty to co-operate with social services departments. Community health practitioners will be required to become involved in identifying and assessing need in order to assist social services and determine whether or not the child is suffering, or is likely to suffer, significant harm. There has been an emphasis in the new Act on greater collaboration and joint planning between health and social services which should begin to have a major effect on community health care planning. Nurses may have an important contribution to make about gaps in the service, the quality of the service and the demand in their area. They may be asked to give references for child minders, or to give training to carers in the social services or education departments. In particular, child care nurses, nurses working in A and E (accident and emergency) departments, and community nurses have a responsibility to participate in the design and implementation of services for the care of children. Nurses can be in the valuable position of being the first to be able to alert others to the position of a child in need.

Local authority child care

The local authority works with other authorities such as housing, education and health to provide a range of facilities for child care, including residential homes, fostering and adoption services, day nurseries, and family centres for families with children showing emotional or behavioural problems, or abuse. They provide therapeutic intervention that may be intensive practical help and support, and may be residential or day-based.

Residential care facilities: residential care includes residential children's homes run by the social services department, hospitals, nursing homes, mental nursing homes, secure accommodation and schools. A change introduced by the Act has been that any health authority that provides accommodation for a child for at least three months must notify the child's local social services department during that period and on discharge of the child. The social services department has a duty to determine the welfare of the child while being accommodated and take account of each child's health, disability, religion, cultural and linguistic background.

Long-term accommodation for children in need may be in one of the following settings:

a) With foster parents to look after the child in their own home as part of their family. In an effort to encourage the views of the child to be taken into consideration, the Act allows foster parents to be relatives or friends of the family or, as was normal practice, to be people whom the child does not know.

b) In a residential home or an education establishment which may be directly managed by the social services departments, voluntary agencies or by the private sector. The Act stresses the importance of the providers of residential care to safeguard and promote the welfare of children being looked after on their premises. The Act requires the local authority to maintain a register, which must be accessible to the public, of persons and institutions who provide care for children on premises other than domestic premises.

In circumstances deemed to be harmful to the welfare of the child, parental responsibility can be granted to local authorities only by an order of the court. Additionally, where the local authority does acquire parental responsibility for children, the Act imposes duties on the local authority to continue to consult and involve parents in decision-making relating to their children (White *et al.*, 1990). The Act supports the need for continued parental responsibility by recognizing that, although parents may not be physically looking after their children, this should not necessarily exclude parents from continuing to carry out a measure of responsibility for their children.

More specifically, the Act stresses the importance of providing children in long-term placements with a sense of permanence and security, experience of normal family life, access to appropriate education and training for a satisfactory job, and social and emotional support. Moreover, local authorities will now continue to have extensive responsibilities for these young adults at least until they are 21 years of age.

Day nurseries: the social services day nurseries usually take children who are on the Child Protection Register, or use a scale of priorities for admission including children from single-parent families, children with special needs, children from very poor housing or families with severe financial problems. They provide a full-day service for parents who work, and will take young babies. A range of other pre-school services provided by education, health or independently are also available, some of which are for children with special needs. There are new regulations in the 1989 Act that require the local authority, through the social services departments, to facilitate the provision of day care services in the community. These regulations aim to ensure the quality of care for children at a nursery or with a childminder, and require that:

a) Those providing day care and childminding services have a duty to register. There is also a duty on local authorities to keep a register which must be accessible to the public.

b) Childminders will have to register if they look after one or more children under the age of eight. Previous legislation required registration for looking after children under the age of five years.

c) Those providing group day care on non-domestic premises have a duty to register if they look after children under the age of eight for more than two hours a day. Previous legislation required registration for looking after children under school-leaving age.

d) Local authorities have rights of inspection of, and entry to, premises without the warrant previously required. At minimum, the local authority is required to conduct an annual inspection of premises used for day care.

Activity
Find out how many social services day nurseries are in your area and determine the criteria for acceptance of children to the nursery.

Education service: because teachers work closely with children every day, they may become aware of social, emotional, behavioural, or physical problems sooner than others and request the help of specialists who work within the education system.

If a child is having particular difficulties at school – whether due to physical, medical, developmental, intellectual, learning, emotional, or behavioural problems – a statement is made of the child's special educational needs. This involves obtaining a number of assessments from professionals involved with the child, including a doctor, a social worker, a teacher, a psychologist, the parents, and any other significant person who has seen the child, such as a speech or occupational therapist. On the basis of these assessments, a plan for the provision of the child's needs is decided; however, no special educational provision can be given without the parent's permission (Smith, 1989).

Schools psychological service: educational psychologists form the basis of this service. They may observe the child at school, or assess their learning abilities and discuss the child with teachers. They will then make recommendations for remediation, either through the child guidance service, special teaching from peripatetic or remedial teachers, or for the child to attend a special unit or residential school. Educational psychologists will also consult more generally with schools about the management of behaviour problems in the school, the design of remedial programmes, and provide staff support and counselling services.

Educational welfare service: educational welfare officers are concerned mostly with school attendance. It is a legal requirement in Britain that all children between the ages of five and sixteen should attend full-time education. If a child is not attending, the educational welfare officer will know through school attendance records. If there is repeated and extensive poor attendance, the officer will visit the family in order to understand the reason and possible problem. They may take a supportive and therapeutic approach themselves, or work with other agencies, such as social services, child guidance units and the schools psychological service. Educational welfare officers have the legal responsibility to take parents to court for poor school attendance.

Pre-school nurseries: many educational authorities provide a pre-school service for children under the age of five. These may or may not be part of primary schools, but will have a qualified teacher in charge. The nurseries take children on a half-day basis, and gradually increase attendance to four or five half-days just before the child starts school.

Voluntary children's organizations: in addition to the community services described, there are many voluntary organizations that provide services for children and their families. Some of these are national or professional organizations; others may be local. Voluntary professional organizations usually work in close co-operation with the statutory services, and include the NSPCC, the Children's Society, Barnado's, National Children's Homes, and many more. There are also special agencies for fostering and adoption, such as the British Association for Adoption and Fostering, National Fostering Care Association, and Parents for Children.

Summary

Primary health care involves promotion of healthy lifestyles, prevention of ill health and rehabilitation. Health promotion has become a community responsibility with nurses becoming involved in facilitating self-help and community support groups.

The issue of identification and prevention of psychological problems in children involves assessment of family functioning within the community, parenting skills, screening for developmental and behavioural problems and detecting abuse. The community health practitioner works with a network of community services and needs to be aware of the role and function of other professionals offering support and help to families and children. The 1989 Act now places great emphasis on the need for children to be brought up in their own homes and the need to avoid legal action except where necessary to safeguard and promote the welfare of the child.

Further reading

Browne, K., Davies, C., and Stratton, P. (Eds) (1988). *Early Prediction and Prevention of Child Abuse*. Chichester, Wiley.
    An informative book that provides empirical and different theoretical approaches to understanding child abuse in the community.

3 *Children with special needs*

Introduction

Children with special needs are children who require additional help and support at home and/or at school because of problems with their intellectual, physical, or emotional behaviour. The term 'special needs' is used in education in order to identify such children, and to provide appropriate services for their needs during their school life.

The Children Act (1989) has defined that a child is disabled 'if he is blind, deaf or dumb or suffers from mental disorder of any kind or is substantially and permanently handicapped by illness, injury or congenital deformity or such other disability as may be prescribed.'

The diagnosis of disability

'Your baby has spina bifida.' 'Your baby has Down's syndrome.' 'Your child cannot see.' When a baby is born, it is usually a time of happiness and hopefulness; but if there is something wrong with the baby, then parents' expectations, hopes, and happiness can be destroyed by a single statement.

How to tell parents about their baby's disability is a difficult and painful task. While doctors will carry most of the initial responsibility, nurses should be part of that process so they can help the parents to understand the implications. Have you considered in detail what would be good practice when telling parents about their baby's disability? Good liaison between staff is essential to ensure that parents' feelings are managed sensitively. All ward staff who have contact with the parents and child should be aware of what has been, or will be, said.

Grief, anger and disbelief

Health professionals have to be able to cope with the grief, anger, and disbelief that parents will experience. Janet Carr (1988) carried out an interesting study in which mothers' answers to questions about the disclosure of their baby's disability were compared when the child was under six months old and when he or she was 21 years old. Across the

71

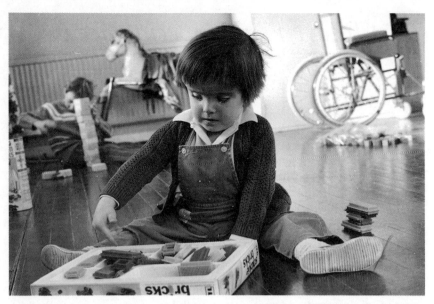

Reprinted by kind permission of MENCAP: Royal Society for Mentally Handicapped Children and Adults.

ten questions asked, 82% of mothers' answers were similar. The most consistent replies were to questions about who gave the news; who was told; whether the news was a shock; whether they would rather have been told later; and whether they had asked for and received a second opinion. Most mothers could still remember the name of the nurse or doctor who broke the news. The greatest difference was on the question, 'Could anything have been done to make the telling easier?', where many mothers changed their opinion, but showing no clear trend. The study found that generally the parents' memories had not become distorted over the years, and that there had been no increase in bitterness or resentment.

Many parents have said in retrospect that they would have liked to have been told together, rather than one being told and having to cope alone until their partner was told. Delays in telling parents who suspect that something is the matter can create immense feelings of anxiety; nurses may have to pretend nothing is the matter until the doctor has seen the parents, but the parents often realize from non-verbal signals that something is seriously wrong.

Parental reaction to such distressing news will vary dramatically according to their personalities, educational level, and cultural background. They may blame themselves, each other, or the staff; they may become angry or violent; they may retreat into disbelief and keep asking for additional information; they may appear stunned and distant while they try to absorb what has been said. Some may only cry later in the privacy of their own home, or they may demonstrate their grief openly and freely. All parents need the opportunity to talk about their feelings, and to feel safe in expressing their innermost thoughts. This can sometimes distress staff, for example, if they hear parents saying 'I wish he had never been born', or, 'I think he should have been left to die'.

Case study

Kwame was admitted at the age of eight weeks for a hernia repair but while in hospital it was noticed that he was usually un-responsive to events around him. Tests indicated that he was visually impaired but his parents did not appear to absorb the information. They kept misinterpreting his behaviour as 'seeing' and kept demonstrating to the nurses that he was normal. The father repeatedly said that 'Kwame will be better when we get him home'.

The diagnosis of a disability begins a long process through which parents come to terms with what the disability means to them. The uncertainty they can feel can induce great anxiety, and they often need questions answered quickly and accurately. Such questions fall into three main areas:

? Questions about the child's condition, and what it means now and for the future, for example, 'How ill is she?', 'Will she always be like this?', 'What caused it?'

? Questions about themselves as parents of a child with disabilities, for example, 'Why did it happen to us?', 'What should we do?', 'How will we cope?', 'Are we to blame?'

? Questions about the effect on family and friends, for example, 'How do we tell the relatives?', 'What will the other children think?', 'Does my partner know how I feel?'

Such questions cannot be answered quickly, and may need to be considered over and over again. As the process of adjustment involves a complete re-analysis of the family lifestyle and function, the need for continuing support is clear. The feelings experienced by parents can disrupt their normal functioning for a period of time. Several phases have been identified, although not all parents go through each phase, and some oscillate or experience phases together (Blacher, 1984). The framework below is one way of understanding parents' reactions.

Shock phase. This may lead into the total disorganization of emotions and paralysis of action lasting for a few minutes or several days. During this time, parents will need strong emotional support.

Reaction phase. Parents start to demonstrate and express their grief, sorrow, disappointment, anxiety, denial, and anger. The process of reintegration begins, as the parents begin to explore possibilities, and test out and learn about their own feelings. They need someone who will listen and will help them to explore their reactions by suggesting alternative explanations, providing accurate information, and reassuring them that their feelings are not unusual.

Adaptation phase. Here, the parents have understood enough to start to anticipate the future. They might have an area of questioning they want to pursue, and can anticipate problems.

Orientation phase. Parents start to organize, seek help, and look to the future. They can manage day-to-day routines, but are continually re-evaluating the future.

Parents of children with disabilities often feel extreme resentment, questioning why it has happened to them. They may not want the responsibility, or be able to confront their pain, and so decide to voluntarily admit the child into care, or give the child up for adoption. Because this can arouse deep feelings in nursing staff, it is important that parents are supported in finding the best solution for themselves and their family, rather than being influenced or feeling judged by nursing attitudes. The decision to give up a baby is much harder than the decision to keep it. Parents may be in fundamental disagreement about this, which can be extremely painful particularly for the partner who wants to keep the baby. Different cultural attitudes will sometimes determine whose opinion is considered most important in the family. For nurses from a different cultural background, this can engender strong feelings towards the dominant parent.

Case study

Nurses felt torn and upset after a baby girl with spina bifida had recovered from her operation to close her back when the father refused to take the baby home. He explicitly stated that he did not want the child and that he wished she had died during the operation. The mother was already attached to the baby and had spent many hours in the ward cuddling her, but she felt she had to do as her husband insisted. She agreed to give the baby up for adoption and eventually left the ward in tears at her final farewell.

The nurse's role is to provide *non-judgmental* support for the parents while they learn to acknowledge the reality of having a child with disabilities. Telling parents to cheer up or that things will be all right will only create a barrier in communication. Such reassurances are often the result of the nurse being unable to cope personally with the level of distress. Nurses need to be able to share their stress with the ward team, and not to block communication with the parents, who need someone who can accept their despair, shoulder their anger, and answer their questions. The way in which this important phase is handled will either enhance or delay the adjustment the parents make to the crisis they are experiencing. Any suggestion of devaluing the baby or ignoring the parents or not recognizing their feelings can produce intense feelings of anger and resentment towards professionals, and may influence the way parents accept or reject professional help in the future.

Exercise

It is important to prepare yourself for the sudden eventuality of talking to parents about their child's disabilities and the stress they feel. Your role is to listen and give them opportunities to talk, not to take away the pain of their distress. Write down a number of questions and statements that you could use when talking to parents about their feelings about having a child with disabilities. Think of your responses to what they might say. (Suggested answers at end of book.)

Assessment of need

The Children Act requires the nurse to share the responsibility for planning services to meet the needs of children who are disabled through physical, sensory or learning disablement, mental disorders and chronic illness. In the past, assessments of need by different agencies have been undertaken separately and the Act now makes it possible to bring together in one process of assessment of need, assessments for several different services where this is appropriate and in the child's best interest.

This change in legislation intends that parents and children are not subject to a confusing variety of assessment procedures. Similarly, assessment of need should be undertaken in an open manner and involve the child and those caring for the child and other significant persons. This supports the view that the family of a child in need has the right to receive sympathetic support and sensitive intervention in their family life.

As a member of a multidisciplinary team responsible for the welfare of children who are disabled, health professionals may be required to give advice, guidance and counselling to families, social services departments and other agencies and most importantly to facilitate the development of preventative health services. In partnership with other agencies, nurses will be required to participate in the provision of care for children in day and long-term care and assist in the training of those caring for children.

Telling the parents: guidelines for nurses

When telling parents about the diagnosis of disability nurses should consider the following:

- parents should be told together if possible
- parents should be asked whether they have any particular suspicions or concerns about the child
- parents should be informed as soon as possible after diagnosis
- there should be time to talk with parents and support their distress at the time of disclosure
- parents should feel free to express their sadness and cry
- parents should be encouraged to ask questions about the disability
- staff involved should be clearly identified and named
- all staff should know what has been said to the parents and how the information was received

Children with learning difficulties

Over the years, the terminology used to describe children with learning difficulties has changed, partly to offset the stigma and perjorative nature of words such as 'retarded', 'subnormal' or 'backward'. The current terminology is concerned with the child's level of functioning.

Before the Education Act (1981) children were categorized so they could be allocated to the special school provision most suitable to their educational needs. The school system included a range of special schools for children with mild to severe learning difficulties. The difficulty of categorizing children occurs at the transition point, or when the child has varying skills and degrees of ability (Forness and Hecht, 1988). The Education Act (1981) introduced a new system of defining children's abilities and identifying their special educational needs so that the provision was suited to the child, rather than the child to the provision. At the same time, integration within schools was introduced so that children of differing abilities were educated together, but with differing levels of special help to meet their particular needs. Gradually, over the past ten years, special schools for children with mild learning difficulties have been closed, and only those for moderate to severe learning difficulties have remained open.

Exercise
What do you think are the positive and negative reasons for having special schools or for integrating all children?

Children with severe learning difficulties

These children often show severe delays in development or severe mental disability from birth. About 55% of severe learning difficulties can be traced to causes occurring before birth, while 20% are due to perinatal problems; about 10% are due to trauma after the child's birth, for example, traffic accidents. In general, the more severe the problem the more likely it is to be physical in origin.

Problems are often apparent in the child's delayed language development and physical milestones. Developmental testing during the first few years of life can start to build a picture of the child's pattern of development, and identify whether there is a general and severe delay across all abilities. Sometimes the pattern is confused when children show islets of abilities – for example, excellent drawing ability or a good memory for patterns – but unless this is reflected in their thinking and language skills, then that special ability will remain an isolated function.

The child's level of language development will be one important way of determining ability. A child with some language, even though it is severely delayed, is easier to communicate with and to understand. The level of physical disability associated with the mental disability will also affect the child's ability to communicate effectively.

Psychological testing can provide an estimate of the child's general intellectual level. The mean ability in the general population is an intelligence quotient (IQ) of 100, but children with severe learning difficulty are considered to have IQs below 50. At this level the IQ becomes rather meaningless, and it is more useful to observe the child's skills and attempt to assess what he or she will be able to do independently. Observing the child's ability in the following areas is helpful in understanding their overall level of development, and for identifying the areas of need and learning:

- Self-help skills: for example, helping in washing and dressing, toileting, eating, and mobility.
- Socialization: for example, the level and type of play, social skills, and social awareness.
- Communication: for example, language, writing skills, and number awareness.

Children with severe learning difficulties, in hospital, have the same needs for company, stimulation and play as any other child. They need the support and presence of their parents like any other children and may also have strong feelings they have difficulty coping with; they can feel as frightened, angry, unhappy, and lonely as any other child, but may not be able to express them so easily through words. Sometimes their feelings of fear may erupt as chronic distress and difficult behaviour because their fears have not been recognized or no-one has been able to explain what is happening. A ten-year-old may be expressing the understanding and fears of a two-year-old. While it is possible to hold, contain, and comfort a two-year-old, it can be far more difficult with a ten-year-old who is lashing out in despair.

For this reason, it is important to gain as much information about the child as possible on admission. The parents should be able to give a good picture of how he or she behaves, and how they manage at home. In order not to distress the child unduly, the parents should be

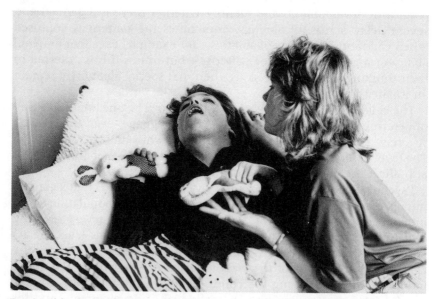

Reprinted by kind permission of MENCAP: Royal Society for Mentally Handicapped Children and Adults.

engaged in the nursing process so they can mediate the necessary nursing activities. The nurse will need to be aware of the child's view of him or herself. He may be aware he is a 'big boy', and will not want to be treated like a little child – even though his feelings and behaviour reflect the infant inside. It will help if his choice of activities and play on the ward are not limited to infant materials and toys.

The adolescent with severe learning difficulties may have similar preoccupations to other teenagers – clothes, make-up and pop stars. They may be concerned about privacy and personal exposure of their bodies, particularly if they have been trained to show modesty. Alternatively, they may have no modesty at all, and may inappropriately expose themselves without realizing the effect on other children and families on the ward.

Children with severe learning difficulties are unable to amuse themselves to the same extent as children of average ability. When left unattended, they will often sit and do nothing because they have poor motivation and little ability to initiate or persevere with activities, or to explore or understand the environment. They need to be shown and helped to experience their surroundings.

Self-stimulatory behaviours are common in these children, who may excessively masturbate, rock, head-bang, or head-shake. They may show self-mutilating behaviour like biting their hands or pulling their hair, and this may be related to the amount of attention they receive. It is important not to go to the child only when he or she is doing these activities. They may need a lot of attention and stimulation to prevent them from lapsing into self-mutilation when unoccupied.

Disorders associated with severe learning difficulties

About one-third of children with severe learning difficulties have a non-progressive brain lesion associated with cerebral palsy, spina bifida, or some other injury. Infections like meningitis also contribute to this figure. About 10%–15% of children with severe learning difficulties are undiagnosed. This can cause great stress to parents, who never understand what has caused their child's disability, and who may spend many years searching for an answer.

Down's syndrome

About 25% of children with learning difficulties have a chromosome disorder, and most of these are diagnosed as Down's syndrome. These children generally function in the upper range of severe learning difficulties, although some show moderate and mild learning difficulties. In a long-term follow-up study, Carr (1988) demonstrated that over the course of the first ten years there was a mean reduction in IQ of approximately 35 points. Some children with Down's syndrome are able to learn to read. Carr found that of 45 twenty-one-year-olds, 45% with Down's syndrome could read with a mean reading accuracy of seven years eight months. As Down's syndrome is an easily identifiable disability that is usually diagnosed at birth, parents are able to link into support networks and services at an early stage in the child's life. There is extensive knowledge and experience about looking after these children and how to help them to develop to their maximum potential.

In recent years, the emphasis on early intervention at home with parents, and later with specialist educational help, indicates that the ability of children with Down's syndrome can improve with structured learning experiences. One study has described how a specialist health visitor provided a home-based service of regularly visiting families who had children with Down's syndrome every six weeks from birth to two years. A short, practical training period of six weeks was found to be adequate for children up to 18 months, but more specialized training was required for older children. Evaluation of the service indicated that parental satisfaction was very high, and that the children progressed favourably (Cunningham *et al.*, 1982a). In a later study, when the family health visitors carried out the home-visiting intervention, the results were less satisfactory. Health visitors who did not have a specialist role and who carried a normal caseload were unable to maintain the intensive visiting, and parental satisfaction was not so great (Cunningham *et al.*, 1982b).

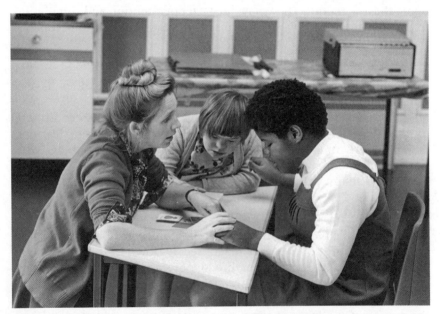

Reprinted by kind permission of MENCAP: Royal Society for Mentally Handicapped Children and Adults.

Home-visiting programmes are also available in the community, with educational psychologists or health visitors carrying out Portage Schemes with parents designed to enhance their child's developmental abilities by teaching the child new skills in small stages. Each stage is reduced to small steps so parents can feel a sense of achievement as their child makes gradual progress. The programme identifies behavioural objectives for the child in five areas of development: infant stimulation, socialization, language, self-help, and cognitive and motor skills. There is a developmental checklist for the parents to fill in and progressively work through. The teaching style is based on behavioural learning theory, and is very systematic, with detailed observation of the child's present behaviour, a definition of each learning objective, and the steps in the teaching process necessary to achieve that objective (Shearer and Shearer, 1972).

Autism

Autism is a rare condition; the prevalence rate in the population is about 10 per 10,000 children (Gillberg, 1990). There is no cure for autism, although outcome is variable. Just under 10% can do well in adult life, i.e. those who have an IQ of over 70 and some communicative speech by the age of five years, while 60% grow up to be totally dependent on their parents in all respects (Gillberg, 1991).

Children with autism often look normal but may have severe impairment of language and communication skills, as well as of social relationships. They have rigid and inflexible thought processes, often expressed in rituals and obsessional or repetitive behaviour. The onset of autism is usually before 36 months of age. Over half of these children show severe learning difficulties, while a small number will function in the average range. A primary symptom of the disorder is the child's lack of awareness of the feelings and behaviour of others. Autistic children may show attachment to their parents, but patterns of eye contact are unusual and abnormal. Communication usually does not include gestures or non-verbal signs. Most do not learn to talk, but if they do, single words or simple phrases are used. A few children learn to speak in sentences, but have difficulty understanding the rules for using language in everyday situations. They often repeat what is said to them (echolalia).

The play of autistic children is unusual in that they are unable to play with toys representing real-life objects. For example, cars will be turned upside down and the wheels spun rather than played with as 'cars'. They may also show rigid obsessional patterns of activity whereby, for example, all objects are put in a special place, paper is torn repeatedly into thin strips, or objects are placed in defined patterns that are not allowed to be disturbed. Autistic children are often upset by any change in routine, and may become extremely distressed.

The cause of autism is not yet known but there have been two main avenues of research in attempting to understand the basic psychological functioning of autistic children. Peter Hobson and his group have developed a theory that the social and communication problems these children have are the result of a basic inability to perceive others' mental states and to interpret feelings and emotions from expressions – an affective disorder (Hobson, 1988). Uta Frith and her group, on the other hand, propose a cognitive deficit theory that is based on the view that autistic children are unable to attribute beliefs and thoughts to others (Baron-Cohen *et al.*, 1986). Normal children are able to understand that people think and have knowledge; they can predict and explain others' behaviour by attributing it to thought processes. If autistic children lack this ability, they are unable to make sense of the social world or to communicate with others (Baron-Cohen, 1989). These two theories provide possibilities for empirical study of the thought processes of autistic children and may lead to important clinical guidelines for understanding and intervention.

Parents require specialist help to learn how to manage their autistic children. They are socially immature and can exhibit extremely difficult and disruptive behaviour. As well as needing constant care and supervision, tantrums, screaming fits, lack of fear, unawareness of danger, destructiveness, and resistance to change can make their care very demanding and wearing. Special educational provision is also needed, and special schools for autistic children are available.

Howlin and Rutter (1987) carried out a long-term controlled study into the effects of a home-based treatment package using behaviour modification principles to teach new behaviour and eliminate unwanted behaviour problems; techniques to foster language skills; and psychological support for the families. This study of 16 high-level autistic boys showed that a six-month treatment programme could effect changes in social competence, language usage, and behaviour problems, but that the effects were not so marked over 18 months. The sample of children studied were of the higher-ability range with no other identifiable handicaps, and so this level of improvement could not necessarily be expected from a more handicapped group.

Mild learning difficulties

Children with mild learning difficulties are often hard to identify. They may show difficulties with all learning and always be slow; they may take much longer than normal children to learn to read and write. They need repeated opportunities to learn new information, and it has to be presented in a simple and structured way; they may also show uneven patterns of ability.

Because many children who suffer emotional or social deprivation at home demonstrate the same difficulties, some people view mild learning difficulties as an environmental rather than a physical problem. But the picture is not as simple as that. This is a mixed group of children with problems of differing aetiology. Children with problems of concentration and attention fall into this group, as this interferes with the ability to learn. Children who show behaviour problems and are aggressive or non-compliant can also fail to learn, as they do not respond to the incentives presented by the teacher for good behaviour.

The fact that a child has mild learning difficulties is unlikely to affect the nurse's management of the child. Problems may occur when attempting to explain something to a child or when information is required from a child but this is more to do with communication skills, and using language and concepts that are understood (Fraser and Rao, 1991).

Specific learning difficulties

Children of average intellectual ability who have specific problems with reading and writing are often considered to have dyslexia. They have trouble with spelling, and often show reversals in letter orientation or letter sequences in words (Hornsby, 1984). Dyslexia has received a lot of attention in recent years as many dyslexic children used to be misdiagnosed as having mild learning difficulties, and so were treated as if they were less able than they were.

Children with dyslexia may be labelled as failures in school when in fact they are very able children with a specific learning difficulty. Their oral work may be excellent, but as much of schoolwork is based on reading and writing, the fact that they are learning by listening, and can tell the teacher all the answers, may be missed in a busy and overcrowded classroom. Early identification is necessary so that specialist and appropriate help can be offered. (M. J. Snowling [1991] presents a comprehensive review of the literature and research in this field.)

Physical disabilities

Physical disabilities can affect a child's mobility, hand co-ordination, language, and physical appearance. Physical disability may or may not be associated with learning difficulties and intellectual delay. When this does occur, the children are considered to be multiply disabled, and present a number of problems that need to be managed at home and at school.

When considering the needs of the child with physical disabilities and their family, health professionals should have the following questions at the back of their minds.

● *How independently mobile is the child? How important is this to the parents?*
Children with cerebral palsy, spina bifida, or congenital physical deformities can all present with differing degrees of immobility. Some children are confined to wheelchairs and will never achieve independent mobility; others may manage to walk although always remain clumsy and poorly co-ordinated. Parents often feel it is essential for their child to learn to walk, as this provides the child with some level of independence and freedom of movement, although with the new developments in powered wheelchairs, many wheelchair-bound children can find a great sense of achievement and control.

● *Is any special physical therapy being offered to the child? How often does this occur? Are the parents involved in the exercises?*
Support from physiotherapists and occupational therapists is necessary for physically handicapped children and their parents in order to learn how best to support the children physically and to encourage appropriate movements. The children require a lot of handling, cuddling, and general movement to become aware of their bodies; they also need slow, careful handling to help them feel secure. Many parents become highly involved in extensive exercise programmes with their children, which take up a large part of each day and require extensive commitment and energy.

● *What does the child do all day at home or when he or she is home from school? How aware are the parents of the child's need for stimulation and support in play?*
If left alone, children with severe physical disabilities are unable to move around to see what is happening, or to see things from a different perspective. They are completely dependent on adults helping them; they are not able to play without toys being brought and demonstrated; if their movements are extremely limited, they need to be shown how to play and to use their skills for the maximum effect. If unattended, such children are often unable to amuse themselves, and so can either become vocally demanding, or sit passively, becoming less and less motivated or interested in their surroundings. In addition to their physical disabilities, the development of a passive attitude to life often compounds any learning difficulties such children may have (Brinker and Lewis, 1982). Television is often used as a time-filler and entertainment for these children, but it is important for the child to

take an active part in family life and to participate in as many activities and tasks as possible. For example, if there is room for the wheelchair in the kitchen, it is far more valuable for the child to be in the kitchen while supper is being prepared, being talked to, than to be left alone in the other room in front of the television. Parents need to develop a directive interactional pattern in order to stimulate responses from their handicapped child (Wassermand *et al.*, 1985).

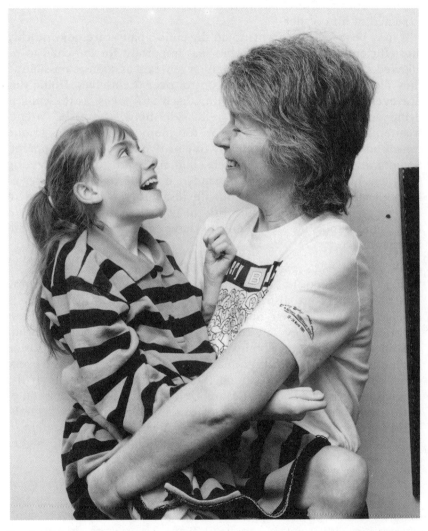

Reprinted by kind permission of MENCAP: Royal Society for Mentally Handicapped Children and Adults. Photographer: Peter Trulock.

● *Are the parents encouraging the child to be as independent as possible in everyday self-help skills? Are they aware of the child's need to exert influence and control?*

Parents may find the physical effort of caring for their child draining on both their energy and emotional resources. There are often difficulties with continence training and other self-help skills such as washing, feeding, and dressing, which are very time-consuming. The effort invested in these basic caring skills sometimes means the parents feel there is little time left for playing with or stimulating their child. They may feel the daily chores can be managed better if they are made into a regular routine; the child then learns what to expect and what is expected of him or her.

It may be faster for parents to do the child's daily-care tasks quickly and efficiently for him or her, but it is important for the child to be allowed and encouraged to do as much self-care as soon as possible so they feel and develop a sense of control over themselves. Doing this however, adds to the amount of time each task takes, as the child is being encouraged to learn as well as to finish the task. Parents frequently find they cannot take on too many teaching roles at one time, and may concentrate on only one or two areas of development. Sometimes they feel sorry for their child and want to do everything for them, but this only fosters dependence and leads to difficulties as the child grows older. Children with disabilities will work hard to achieve a sense of mastery, and with the growth of microtechnology it is becoming possible for them to have greater self-control and independence.

● *What is the child's intellectual level of development?*

While a high proportion of children with cerebral palsy have learning difficulties, there are also a number with average or above-average intellectual ability. Their opportunity to communicate and express themselves may be severely curtailed by their physical disabilities but this does not mean their brains are not working, locked away inside bodies they cannot control. With all physically disabled children every effort should be made to extend their communication skills to the maximum via any aid possible. Many children with physical disabilities with normal intellectual ability can cope with mainstream schools, with additional support for their physical needs and computers to facilitate communication and written work. Some progress to higher education.

● *If the child has language and communication difficulties, what support and advice is being offered to aid communication at home?*

When a child's physical disability is compounded with severe communication difficulties it can be difficult for parents, friends, and relatives to estimate how much the child can understand. It is easy to under- or over-estimate the child's intellectual ability. Parents may need help in developing simple communication systems to enable the child to express its needs and desires, such as the use of signs and symbols. A speech and language therapist can help parents to develop and learn the system, and teach the child how best to make their needs understood.

> **Activity**
> Identify and locate the network of services that exists for a child with cerebral palsy in the area where you work or where you live. Remember to contact health, education and social services, plus voluntary agencies and self-help groups.

Sensory disabilities

Visual disability

Visual disability can vary in its severity. It can also occur in the context of other mental and physical disabilities. Children with visual disabilities are usually categorized into 'partially sighted' or 'blind' groups, and once registered can receive special services and provision.

The parents of babies with visual disabilities often need a great deal of special help in order to understand and know their baby; it can be very difficult for a parent to relate to a baby who does not respond with the normal signs and gestures of attachment: a blind baby will not smile in response to the parents' smile; it will not look at them or try to engage them in contact. Understandably, the parents feel upset when they look into their baby's unseeing eyes. The blind baby will have a restricted range of behaviours, and parents need to be alert to the special signals their baby is showing. Increased hand movements or smiles in response to sounds of the parents' voices can occur when no one is looking, and these signs of recognition are often missed. Rather than show animation and physical response, blind babies may go still when approached in order to listen to what is happening.

The normal development sequences are also affected. A blind child's attempts to walk are likely to be delayed, and many blind children never crawl. Similarly, language development may be delayed. Some blind children exhibit repetitive self-stimulatory behaviours like head-banging, eye-poking, and rocking, which are often to do with social isolation. Increasing the level of stimulation and contact with such children, and encouraging them to participate fully in activities and to stretch their abilities will help overcome these difficulties.

The educational needs of children with visual disabilities include not only teaching them to read and write and understand mathematical concepts, but also to train them in posture, locomotion, orientation, and navigation skills, that is, mobility. As blind children do not have guide dogs, this includes the use of a cane as a mobility aid. Blind children also need to gain confidence in their physical skills in informal ways, like climbing, swinging, jumping, and balancing. At home, the blind child should be encouraged to walk around the house independently, learning about the environment through experiencing it.

Technology is aiding many partially sighted and blind children to be taught to read and write through conventional methods, rather than Braille. Closed-circuit television magnifies written work beyond the level of optical magnification, allowing the child to read normal-sized books. It is now also possible for blind children to store and retrieve information using microcomputers to support their educational experience at school, and later in their working life.

Hearing impairment

A large number of children suffer intermittent hearing loss due to the build-up of fluid in the middle ear. Thirty per cent of children under the age of two have been found to have middle ear disorders (Reichman and Healey, 1983), and in a survey of London nursery children, Shah (1981) found evidence of unsuspected middle ear infection in 35% of the children. The critical time for adverse effects is during the first three years of life. Hearing loss during this time will create a delay in language development rather than a deviant pattern. Active medical management of the hearing loss will resolve the problem rapidly, but if it continues undetected or intermittently it can have serious implications for the child's academic performance later in school.

Deafness has much greater implications for the development of the child. It creates problems with socialization and discipline as parents are less able to use rationalization and explanation in the control of their child's behaviour. Deaf children therefore may become frustrated and have more temper-tantrums in their early years. The young deaf child has difficulties understanding temporal and time relations: talking about the past, present, and future, and learning to anticipate events can all be lost in the child's early experience.

Difficulties occur also for deaf children in learning to communicate with their parents. Language may be severely delayed or distorted by the hearing impairment, and the child may need special training to learn how to regulate tone, volume, and pitch. Microcomputers can give children visual feedback of the sound patterns they generate when they speak, which can help them to regulate their speech production. There has been much controversy about what kind of communication system should be taught to deaf children, whether it should be primarily aural or should use hand signing. The professionals who use aural methods give the children hearing aids, and all communication is via high-quality sound amplification, in order to teach them to listen and use any residual hearing they have.

Figure 3.1 *Makaton signs*

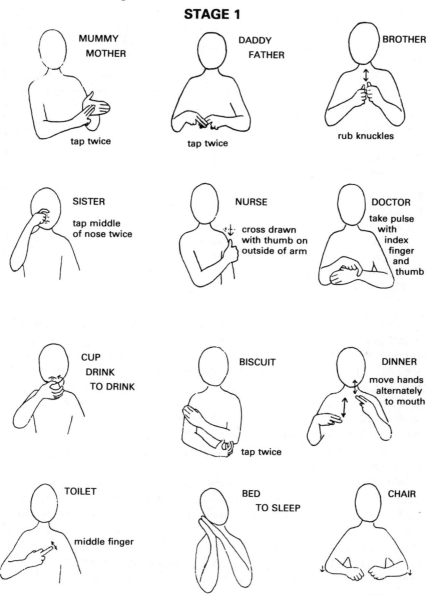

From Makaton Vocabulary Development Project. Reproduced with permission.

Figure 3.2 *Blissymbolics*

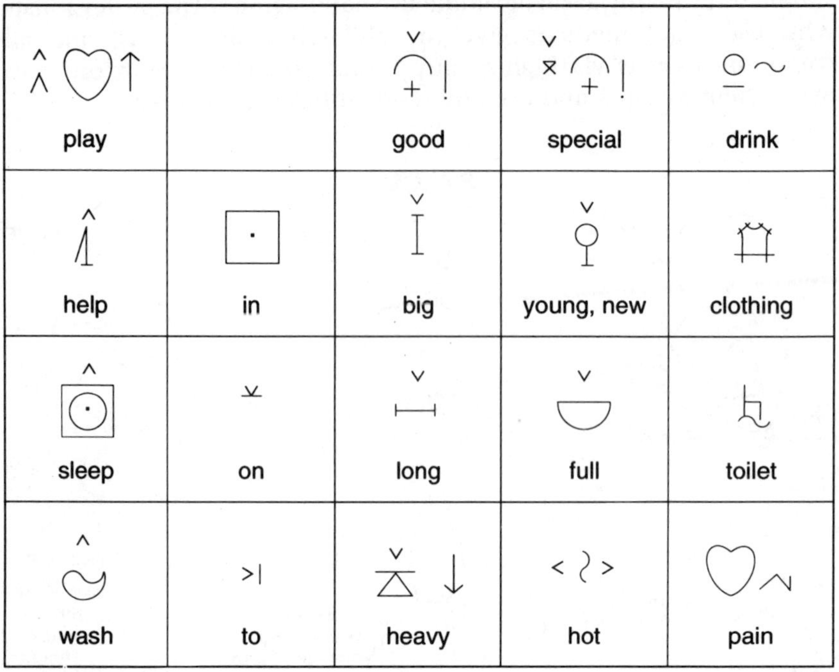

⌃ ♡ ↑ ⋀ play		⌃ ⌒ ¦ + ! good	⌃ ⤫ ⌒ ¦ + ! special	○ ∼ ⊖ drink
⌃ ⌁ help	▢ · in	⌄ Ĭ big	⌄ ○ ⌁ young, new	⌂ clothing
⌃ ▣ ⊙ sleep	⤓ on	⌄ ⊢—⊣ long	⌄ ⌣ full	♄ toilet
⌃ ⌣ wash	>¦ to	⌄ △ ↓ heavy	< ? > hot	♡ ∧ pain

From Blissymbolics Communication Resource Centre (UK), South Glamorgan Institute of Higher Education.

If the child has a considerable hearing loss, a manual system usually accompanies speech. These include hand signs and signals that are used to supplement or replace speech sounds. There are many different sign systems; the one used most commonly in Britain is the British Sign Language, which is a language in its own right and can be supplemented by finger spelling. Makaton is another communication system that uses signs, speech and graphic symbols for use across a wide range of communication and learning difficulties. Cued speech is a manual system designed to supplement speech rather than replace it, and aids in lip-reading.

Whether to emphasize oral methods or to use manual methods can depend on the severity of the hearing loss. An oral method allows the handicapped child to integrate more easily into the hearing community, but it is also associated with low achievement; manual systems may ease learning skills initially, but can isolate the deaf child with other deaf children and the few adults that know the system. Most specialists now advocate a total communication approach that uses signs to supplement oral methods.

Families with special needs children

Research studies are now identifying the areas of support required in some families and can help guide health professionals in how best to target services. Many research studies have been carried out on variables related to poor outcome in families of children with disabilities, but not all families fail to cope: there is a wide range of adaptation from successful to maladaptive. A recent study attempted to discover which aspects of stress and family functioning are most related to outcome (Sloper *et al.*, 1991). It also examined factors related to coping and good outcome, rather than just focusing on variables related to poor outcome. This more positive orientation is necessary to understand the qualities that enable families to cope despite terrible circumstances and experiences. This excellent and comprehensive study examined in detail:

a) the child's characteristics associated with Down's syndrome
b) the family characteristics
c) the parental and family resources
d) the coping factors.

These were related to outcome measures of the parents' level of satisfaction with life and with the level of stress or malaise that they were experiencing. Parental stress was measured on a 24-item checklist of psychosomatic symptoms, and parental satisfaction with life included a range of measures compiled by the authors. Tables 3.1 and 3.2 show the variables that were significantly associated with the outcome measures for both mothers and fathers.

For the mothers, the variable most strongly associated with their perceived satisfaction of life was their neuroticism score: the lower the level of neuroticism, the higher their level of satisfaction. Seven other variables were also related to better outcome. These were higher levels of family cohesion, better marital relationship, high child self-sufficiency, lower child excitability, both parents being employed, and the greater use of practical coping strategies. For fathers, the variable most strongly associated with perceived satisfaction with life was the marital relationship: the better the marriage, the higher the satisfaction.

There was a significant difference between the mothers and fathers on the level of stress experienced, with mothers experiencing far higher stress. The variable most highly associated with this was their neuroticism score, but in addition, high rates of child behaviour problems, lack of a car, and high rates of wishful thinking used as a coping strategy were found to be related to high rates of stress. For the fathers, the variables most strongly related to stress were neuroticism scores and marital relationship.

Table 3.1 *Variables significantly associated with outcome measures in univariate analyses for mothers (from Sloper* et al., *1991)*

Descriptor variable	Perceived satisfaction with life	Malaise
(a) *Child variables*		
Mental age +	**	**
IQ +	*	*
Academic abilities +	***	**
Self-sufficiency +	***	*
Behaviour problems −	***	***
Social life +	***	*
Excitability −	*	n.s.
Supervision needs −	**	*
Caretaking needs −	*	n.s.
(b) *Family characteristics*		
Mother in employment +	*	**
Financial problems	***	***
Housing adequacy −	*	**
Father in employment +	*	n.s.
Social class +	n.s.	**
Type of neighbourhood +	n.s.	*
Car ownership +	n.s.	**
(c) *Parental and family resources*		
Neuroticism −	***	***
Marital relationship +	***	*
Family conflict −	***	***
Locus of control +	*	**
Family cohesion +	***	***
Family expression +	***	**
Active recreational orientation +	***	**
Organization +	***	*
Amount of social support +	***	***
Adaptation to child +	***	***
Sibling behaviour problems −	**	***
Life events strain −	*	***
No. of life events −	n.s.	**
Illness in last year −	*	***
Hospitalization in last year −	n.s.	**
(d) *Coping factors*		
Practical coping +	**	**
Wishful thinking −	***	***
Stoicism +	*	n.s.
Passive acceptance −	*	n.s.
Seeking emotional social support +	n.s.	*

Significance levels: ***$p < 0.001$; **$p < 0.01$; *$p < 0.05$.
+/− = direction of relationship.

Table 3.2 *Variables significantly associated with outcome measures in univariate analyses for fathers (from Sloper et al., 1991)*

Descriptor variable	Perceived satisfaction with life	Malaise
(a) *Child variables*		
Mental age +	*	n.s.
Academic abilities +	*	n.s.
Self-sufficiency +	**	**
Behaviour problems −	**	***
Social life +	**	n.s.
Supervision needs −	*	n.s.
Gender − female +	*	n.s.
(b) *Family characteristics*		
Financial problems −	**	*
Father in employment +	n.s.	**
(c) *Parental and family resources*		
Neuroticism −	***	***
Marital relationship +	***	**
Family conflict −	**	**
Locus of control +	*	n.s.
Family cohesion +	***	***
Family expression +	**	n.s.
Active recreational orientation +	n.s.	*
Organization +	**	n.s.
Amount of social support +	**	**
Adaptation to child +	***	***
Sibling behaviour problems −	*	*
Life events strain −	***	n.s.
Illness in last year −	n.s.	*
(d) *Coping factors*		
Wishful thinking −	n.s.	***
Passive acceptance −	***	n.s.
Seeking emotional social support +	**	n.s.

Significance levels: ***$p < 0.001$; **$p < 0.01$; *$p < 0.05$.
+/− = direction of relationship.

This study provides important guidelines for community service provision for families with handicapped children. The analysis of the effect on the mothers indicates that some women have a personal vulnerability to stress, which may be a key to identifying which families are less likely to be able to cope with having a handicapped child. Severity of the child's disability and behaviour problems was also related to poor maternal functioning, and this may identify the need for family and behavioural intervention with the child's behavioural difficulties.

A positive attitude to the child does not in itself remove the stressful effects of behaviour problems, but it does enable the mother to view them as less central to the parents' relationship with their child. Attention should therefore be given to the mother–child relationship, and to interpreting causes of behaviour problems in order to help parents view their child in a more positive light (Cunningham and Davis, 1985).

Families who are experiencing socio-economic difficulties also experience high levels of stress, and so the provision of material resources could be an important factor in ameliorating stress.

Coping strategies also have an effect on the mothers' reactions to potential stressors. This study did not examine the effect of coping strategies over time, and it is not clear whether poor coping strategies are related to increasing problems within the family. Poor strategies may also be the outcome of parents having tried to cope but failed, and then giving up. Community services to families should therefore address the issues of early identification of behaviour problems, problem-solving strategies, and enabling parents to obtain easy access to service support.

The mothers who are most likely to be able to cope with their child's behaviour problems without risk to their own health are those who have good adjustment to the child; have suffered few significant life events in the preceding year; are employed; and are from a non-manual social class. Life events include important occurrences to the family, for example, birth of a baby, loss of a job, bereavement, etc. Services to families should take account of family events that may be unrelated to the child, but can adversely affect the family, for example, financial and employment difficulties.

The effects on mothers and fathers of having a child with Down's syndrome are very different. The child's characteristics are not the main sources of stress for fathers as they are for mothers. Fathers are far more affected by events external to the child, for example, unemployment. The quality of the marital relationship is also more important, and may act as an important resource for fathers. There is no theoretical connection between the sources of stress and coping factors for fathers, but there is an important moderating effect of personality in how fathers react to potential stressors, as there is in mothers.

This study found no significant relationships between outcome measures and social support. It appears that social support is mediated by factors internal to the parent and family, as the parents' personality characteristics and marital satisfaction appear to be more important. The relationship between coping and social support may be interactive, with better copers having more social support and more social support facilitating coping (Friedrich *et al.*, 1985). Intervention should examine how social support is mediated and attempt to influence parents' access to and use of support.

It is clear that multidimensional models are needed to identify factors that relate to risk, and to distinguish families that are adaptive or maladaptive. Interventions that target only one aspect of family functioning, like the child's behaviour, are less likely to succeed than those which focus on broader aspects. It is interesting to speculate whether providing support services to enable mothers to cope better and perhaps go out to work could have a positive effect on their mental health, and consequently on their marriage. This in turn could positively affect the father's response to stress.

The nurse's role with children with special needs

Nurses have a significant role to play in helping parents to learn how to manage their children so they become less dependent, and to teach them necessary skills to reduce the level of disability. Figure 3.3 demonstrates the sequence of procedures implied by two different approaches to parent support.

The care approach involves an analysis of the tasks required in caring for a child with disabilities, including observation of how the parent carries out the activities, for example, how to move and position the

Figure 3.3 *Two approaches to parent support*

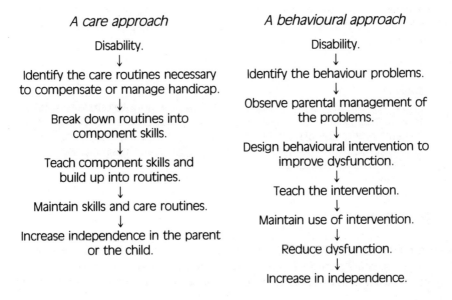

A care approach	A behavioural approach
Disability.	Disability.
↓	↓
Identify the care routines necessary to compensate or manage handicap.	Identify the behaviour problems.
↓	↓
Break down routines into component skills.	Observe parental management of the problems.
↓	↓
Teach component skills and build up into routines.	Design behavioural intervention to improve dysfunction.
↓	↓
Maintain skills and care routines.	Teach the intervention.
↓	↓
Increase independence in the parent or the child.	Maintain use of intervention.
	↓
	Reduce dysfunction.
	↓
	Increase in independence.

child, or home tracheostomy care. The aim is to build competency in the parent. The tasks can be broken down into simple steps, each of which can be taught and tailored to the individual parent and child.

The behavioural approach involves teaching parents how to manage their child's behaviour more effectively. For example, bowel management of children with spina bifida often causes concern. Approximately 25% of children with myelomeningocele can develop continence, and another third are able to significantly improve their bowel control with basic behavioural management techniques used in the home. One study, in a nursery of 27 children with cerebral palsy aged two-and-a-half and four years, found that 97% became reliably dry in five weeks with simple and consistent toilet training management (Shaw, 1990). Many children with disabilities have severe sleep problems, which can dramatically compound the stress on the parents, but basic sleep management advice can have very beneficial effects on the level of sleep disturbance. It is important for parents not to give up on basic management skills. They will need support and help in what to do and how to implement it.

Language and communication development is also a vital area of intervention in many families with children who have special needs. A large number of early-language intervention programmes exist, many of which can be applied without specialist knowledge. Helping parents to develop their child's language skills has moved away from highly structured learning programmes to those that are more flexible and treat the child as an active learner. Activities that promote verbal spontaneity in social interactions are now considered to be important, as well as pre-verbal communication and symbolic play skills. Nurses can play a significant role in supporting and encouraging parents to talk with their children, and provide a stimulating and enriching verbal environment.

Exercise

Within the provisions of the Act, children have the right to refuse to submit to a medical examination, assessment or treatment if they are of sufficient understanding to make an informed decision. What is the likely impact of this on your practice and how can you ensure and maintain the confidence and trust of the child?

Summary

Paediatric nurses have frequent contact with children who have special needs through caring for those who have long-term and chronic physical disorders and those who have

mental and physical disabilities. In law, for the first time, children with disabilities are to be treated as children with particular needs and are entitled to the same general level of social services as any other children in need to enable them to live as normal a life as possible (HMSO, 1989). Therefore the health services need to work, co-operating with social services, to identify the needs of children in each area who are disabled through physical, sensory or learning disabilities, mental disorders or chronic illness.

Nurses need to be aware of the range of children's disabilities and the variation in severity. Many of these children's difficulties are compounded by additional behavioural problems and parents often require extensive support and advice on how to cope and manage their child. Nurses are often at the forefront of listening to parents' worries and anxieties about their children and need to be aware of the issues facing these families on a daily basis.

Nurses may be involved at the point of diagnosis of disability or as a long-term carer of the child. Counselling and support may be necessary for the family as well as structured developmental programmes. The development of daily care routines at home can also include managing behavioural and emotional difficulties.

Further reading

Daly, B., Addington, J., Kerfoot, S. and Sigston, A. (1985). *Portage: The importance of parents.* N.F.E.R./Nelson, Windsor.
This book is a collection of articles that provide a good overview of the application of Portage with families and includes work with severely mentally and visually handicapped children and a cross cultural look at work with Asian families. It is practically based and provides detailed description of different projects that have used Portage materials in the home. One section includes several articles on the learning of language skills. It also discusses methods of using Portage to help with family problems.

Griffiths, M. and Russel, P. (1985). *Working Together with Handicapped Children.* Souvenir Press, London.
This book provides a comprehensive view of children's motor, visual and communication disabilities. It also includes specific learning problems, multiple disabilities and emotional and social problems. It looks at issues in assessment, support and remediation.

McCarthy, G. T. (ed.) (1984). *The Physically Handicapped Child.* Faber & Faber, London.
This book has chapters on each of the major physical disabilities and then considers the range of support services that are required to help these children. It provides information on wheelchairs and seating, education and

microtechnology as well as examining the issues facing the older child with physical disabilities i.e. social integration and sexuality.

Nolan, M. and Tucker, I. G. (1981). *The Hearing Impaired Child and the Family*. Souvenir Press, London.
This is a very readable book that describes the effect of a hearing impaired child on family life. It provides a valuable insight to the problems faced by parents for the nurse in community care.

4 Children's behavioural and emotional problems

Introduction

Although behavioural and emotional problems can occur in addition to medical problems, in some instances they are the main reason for the child's admission to hospital. An adolescent who has stopped eating and become anorexic; a child who has tried to commit suicide; a toddler who is failing to thrive; a pre-schooler who will not sleep; or a junior-age child who is soiling and wetting are all examples of children who may be admitted for observation, treatment, or investigation for psychological problems.

Parents of young children often seek practical advice on how to cope with a range of behaviour difficulties, ranging from eating, sleeping, and toileting problems, to managing aggressive and disobedient behaviour. Parents of adolescents worry more about pregnancy, smoking, and drug and alcohol abuse. Concerns about a breakdown in communication with adolescents, the conflict between a desire to control a growing child who still needs protecting but who already has his or her own opinions and attitudes can cause great stress.

Behaviour problems

When caring for ill children, behavioural and emotional problems add another dimension to the nursing role. Such children may not automatically co-operate, often they have not learned what is expected of them, or they don't understand what is happening. They can be fearful or anxious; aggressive and defiant; non-compliant, or depressed and withdrawn.

The nurse has an important role in community health promotion, and knowledge and awareness of the behaviour problems of childhood are a necessary part of understanding the whole child. The community health practitioner may help parents specifically with their child's behaviour problems. Health professionals also need to understand children's behaviour problems in order to complete nursing tasks necessary for the child's well-being. Children show a wide variety of problems, which fall into different categories.

Conduct problems

Children with conduct problems are aggressive, defiant, disobedient, and destructive. They may lie, steal, play truant, and have tantrums. They show difficult behaviour at home and at school, and often fail academically. The older age range may become delinquent. Conduct disorder is far more common in boys than in girls. Children of criminal and alcoholic parents also show a greatly increased risk of the disorder, particularly if the mother is affected (Rutter, 1985). Whether the transmission of conduct disorder is primarily environmental or genetic and biological is not yet clear; however, the strongest correlate is the pattern of poor parental disciplinary practices. Parents of such children are often described as being neglectful, erratic, and harsh in their punishment (Robins, 1991).

Hyperactivity and attention deficit disorder

It is often difficult to determine whether a child is showing hyperactive behaviour or conduct disorder, and there has been much disagreement about clear diagnostic criteria for these disorders. Hyperactivity describes children who show inattentiveness, overactivity, and impulsiveness in *some* situations; hyperkinetic syndrome refers to children who show pervasive hyperactivity in *all* situations. Some children show attention deficit disorder without hyperactivity. In Britain, the prevalence of attention deficit disorder is approximately 1%, while attention deficit disorder with hyperactivity is between 6% and 15%. Hyperkinetic syndrome occurs in 1.7% of boys (Schachar, 1991).

Young children's problems

These include difficulties in sleeping, eating, and toileting; habits like thumb-sucking; and other early management issues of disobedience and temper-tantrums. The prevalence rate of these problems in a central London borough revealed that 15% of pre-school children had mild behaviour problems, 6.2% had moderate problems, and 1.1% had severe problems (Richman *et al.*, 1982). The problems also persist: 63% of three-year-olds were considered to still have behaviour problems one and five years later. The gender of the child also has a significant effect on the persistence rate, as 73% of boys, but only 47% of girls, still had problems at eight years. The most accurate predictor of outcome is the severity of the behaviour problem: the more severe the problem, the more likely it is to persist.

Enuresis

Most children achieve day and night continence by the age of four. They are usually dry by day before they are dry by night. At nearly all ages the prevalence in boys is greater than in girls. Bedwetting is rare in girls after 11 years, and rare in boys after 13 years.

Diurnal enuresis is less common than nocturnal enuresis, and occurs in girls more than in boys. About 2% of five-year-olds are wet in the day once a week or more, although about 8% are wet at least once a month (DeJonge, 1973). In the seven to ten-year age range, only 1% of children have daytime wetting.

Primary enuresis indicates that the child never achieved continence, while secondary enuresis indicates a lapse in continence. Enuresis tends to run in families, and so genetic factors have been implicated.

Encopresis

Children usually achieve faecal continence by the age of three years, but 16% of three-year-olds still show signs of faecal incontinence once a week or more (Richman *et al.*, 1982). By the age of four this has reduced to 3%. By age seven only 1.5% of children still soil, and by ten to eleven years this is down to 0.8% (Bellman, 1966). The types of encopresis are shown in Figure. 4.1.

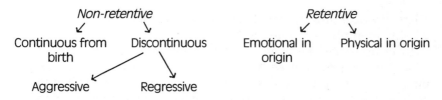

Figure 4.1 *Types of encopresis*

Retentive encopresis is the accumulation of faeces in the colon or rectum resulting in constipation and overflow. It may be physical in nature, e.g., due to anal fissure, or it may be emotional in nature and related to a disturbed parent–child relationship. Coercive or rigid toilet-training, and high levels of anxiety or anger are related to this type of encopresis.

In non-retentive encopresis, that has been continuous from birth, the child has never achieved faecal continence. It is often associated with physical neglect and poor social training. Such children may never have had the opportunity or been taught to use the toilet. Discontinuous encopresis, on the other hand, can be regressive, i.e., due to an acute or continuing stress that causes the child to regress to immature behaviour; or it may be aggressive, as when the child refuses to defecate in the right place or when the parents request it. This can be associated with smearing, and can be characterized by passing motions in unusual and inappropriate places.

Adolescent behaviour problems

The pattern of behaviour disorders changes as children develop into adolescents. Schizophrenia and depression, which are rare before puberty, become more common, while encopresis, enuresis, and childhood behaviour problems become less common. There is a shift in the gender ratio from a higher level of behaviour problems in boys in early childhood, to a higher proportion in girls in adolescence. This is accounted for by an increase in the number of affective disorders in adolescent girls. Alcohol and drug abuse, and anorexia nervosa are also conditions that are uncommon before puberty, except glue- and petrol-sniffing, which occur also in early childhood.

Unresolved childhood conflicts can cause a number of ongoing behaviour problems, for example conduct disorders leading to delinquency, school refusal, attention deficit disorder, plus a number of anxiety states. Drug and substance abuse, in particular, has become a serious problem over the last 20 years.

Drug abuse

There is a clear progression of drug abuse with age, and the mid-teens is a common time for abuse to begin.

Drug users may be experimental, situation, or compulsive. Many adolescents experiment with smoking, alcohol, or marijuana at some time; others may use drugs at parties, while only a small number become habitual users. It is not clear why some adolescents become dependent on drugs. Social pressure can encourage drug use, but probably not dependence. Addiction may be more related to personality characteristics and emotional state. There is a strong correlation

Table 4.1 *Prevalence of drug use in 14 to 16-year-olds (Offord et al., 1987, Ontario Health Study)*

Substance		Boys (%)	Girls (%)
Tobacco	– occasional use	31.1	45.6
	– regular use	15.8	23.4
Alcohol	– occasional use	42.5	48.8
	– regular use	10.6	15.9
Marijuana		13.3	17.6
Hard drugs		5.3	7.5
Inhalants		3.8	4.5

between parental and adolescent smoking. The chances of becoming a teenage smoker are about five times greater in smoking than in non-smoking households (Barker, 1988).

Vicary and Lerner (1986) report results from a longitudinal study that found that early parental conflict over child rearing, and harsh and restrictive parenting was associated with drug use in the teen years. There is also a correlation between drug abuse, delinquency, and school failure, but correlations do not indicate causal relationships, and there may be common factors relating to all three problems.

Anorexia nervosa

This is predominantly found in adolescent girls, although early onset can occur in pre-pubertal boys and girls. The essential feature is a profound aversion to food, leading to serious and sometimes life-threatening weight loss. Symptoms include excessive physical activity

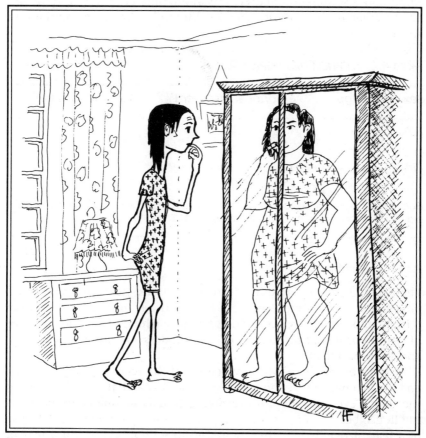

Perception? I know what I look like.

to induce weight loss, depression, amenorrhoea, self-induced vomiting, and laxative abuse. The cause of this disorder is not clear, but certain features are well recognized. Many adolescents have a fear of growing up, and show sexual anxiety by returning to a physically pre-pubertal state. Society's emphasis on slim female figures has also focused attention on women's weight and shape. On a psychological level, the disorder can be seen as a distorted struggle for self-control and autonomy. There are also significant physiological changes, but whether these predate the psychological problems is not yet clear.

Emotional problems

Emotional problems indicate a disturbance in a child's feelings, and also in how they express their feelings. Sometimes this shows itself as a behaviour problem. In one London borough, the prevalence of emotional disorders in children was approximately 5% (Rutter *et al.*, 1970); while in the Ontario Child Health Study, the percentages found are shown in Table 4.2.

Table 4.2 *Ontario Child Health Study*

Sex	Age	Emotional disorder (%)	Somatization (%)
Boys	4–11	10.2	–
	12–16	4.9	4.5
Girls	4–11	10.7	–
	12–16	13.6	10.7

[Somatization was defined as the presence of recurrent, multiple and vague physical symptoms without physical cause (Offord *et al.*, 1987)]

Anxiety problems

These include separation difficulties, panic attacks, fearfulness, phobias, obsessional and compulsive behaviour (rare in children), school refusal, and some psychosomatic problems. Children describe a range of symptoms including nausea, pains, dizziness, sweating, restlessness, and sleep problems.

Anxiety normally leads to avoidance of the feared event or object, and the avoidance reaction can become so strong that it interferes with the child's everyday life, for example they may be unable to go out of the house because of a fear of dogs; they won't go to hospital because of a fear of needles; or they won't go to school because of a fear of separating from their mother. Specific fears and phobias are common among young children, but they decline and change as the child grows older. When a child experiences such severe anxiety that it is converted into a physical symptom, it is called a conversion disorder, for example in symptoms of blindness, paralysis, or mutism.

Exercise
List as many childhood phobias and fears as you can think of.
(Suggested answers at end of book.)

Depressive states

The prevalence rates of pre-pubertal depression vary markedly. Young children aged one to six years show very low rates of major depression, compared to children in the six to twelve year ranges (Kashani *et al.*, 1984). The Isle of Wight study (Rutter, *et al.*, 1970) demonstrated the effect of the pubertal state on the type and incidence of depression. Depressive symptoms were twice as common in pre-pubertal boys, and twice as common in post-pubertal girls. Of the ten to eleven-year-olds from the general population, 13% showed depressed mood. When these children were reassessed at age fourteen to fifteen, over 40% reported feelings of misery and depression (Rutter *et al.*, 1986).

Suicide is often associated with depression, but it is rare before the ages of twelve to fourteen. The rate of suicide and attempted suicide rises sharply during adolescence, although pre-pubertal children can express suicidal thoughts.

Mental illness

The essential feature of psychotic disorders is a distorted or altered sense of reality.

Childhood schizophrenia

Whether schizophrenia occurs before the age of five is open to question, but for many years there has been a confusion in diagnosis between childhood schizophrenia and autism in the pre-school age group. Schizophrenia occurs more commonly after puberty and during late adolescence. The schizophrenic child may have delusions, for example imagining that their thoughts are being controlled from outside their bodies, or that others are always talking about them. They may have hallucinations, as when they imagine they hear voices talking to them. They may also have thought disorders when their thoughts seem to drift between different subjects in an unsystematic way. Their emotional reactions may be flat or inappropriate, and they may show unusual or bizarre bodily movements.

Disintegrative psychoses

Here, normal to near-normal development for the first few years is followed by a loss of social skills and speech, together with a severe disorder of emotions, behaviour, and relationships. The child's intellectual level deteriorates, and they start to show disturbed, overactive, and uncharacteristic behaviour. This is often due to organic brain disease, and may be progressive or non-progressive. Encephalitis, seizures, and lead poisoning have all been identified as non-progressive causes, while degenerative neurological conditions and Aids can lead to the dementing process (Barker, 1988).

Assessing behavioural and emotional problems

Assessing and interviewing the child and family is the first stage in developing a treatment plan. The type of interview will depend on the information that is required, and a flexible approach is necessary. The child can be seen alone or with the family, or the parents can be seen alone. Many therapists prefer to see the family as a group in order to assess the different factors in the child's home life that may be contributing to his or her present emotional or behavioural state.

A series of studies of interviewing techniques was carried out at the Maudsley Hospital, London, to assess the effectiveness of different approaches in eliciting fact and feelings from parents or children referred for psychiatric assessment (Rutter *et al.*, 1981). It was found that an active, structured approach, used sensitively and with the interviewer alert for clues to unusual symptoms, is best for eliciting facts (Cox *et al.*, 1981a). When trying to elicit feelings, the use of open questions, rather than yes or no questions, a low voice, direct requests for the expression of feelings, combined with interpretations and expressions of sympathy, were found to be most helpful (Cox *et al.*, 1981b). Structured interviewing was more effective than relying on spontaneous parental reports of their children's behaviour. Although many different interviewing styles may be used, the following questions provide a useful pattern for investigating children's behaviour problems.

Assessing present experiences and behaviour

● *How often is the problem occurring?*
The frequency of the problem is important in deciding its severity. A three-year-old child may have one tantrum every day, but if they are having five tantrums a day, then the problem is severe. It is also helpful to find out whether the problem occurs at certain times of the day, with certain people, or is situation specific.

● *How extreme is the problem?*
The intensity of the problem is another way of determining its severity. Most children refuse to co-operate at some time, but if the child regularly becomes aggressive or abusive then this indicates an intense problem. Many four-year-olds are fearful of leaving their parents, but if they cling excessively and cry inconsolably for long periods when separated, their anxiety may be considered severe.

● *How long has there been a problem?*
The length of the problem will give an indication of its severity. A child who goes off eating for a couple of days is different from the child who continuously refuses to eat and starts to lose weight.

● *Does the child show other problems?*
Problems often occur together, and the more problems a child has the more worrying the situation becomes. A child may be aggressive occasionally, but if he or she is also overactive, shows poor concentration, and has few friends, then they are likely to have difficulties at school and present a management problem. A seven-year-old who is fearful and withdrawn, has rituals such as only walking on alternate steps on the stairs, has to have the curtains four inches apart at night-time, and also wets the bed, is presenting with significant anxiety symptoms.

● *Are the child's behaviour and emotions appropriate for their developmental level?*
If a child is showing a delay in development, then their general behaviour and emotional control will also be immature. Such children tend to have more behaviour problems, which may need to be managed in the context of their disability or learning difficulty. If the child is of normal development, then immature and uncontrolled behaviour is often a reflection of parental management styles, experiences, or poor opportunities for learning how to behave appropriately.

● *Does the child have any sensory disabilities?*
Many children with poor hearing or intermittent hearing loss appear to be disobedient and unco-operative because they cannot hear what is

being said to them. They can also feel frustrated by their inability to communicate adequately with others, and may be aggressive in their reactions. A child who cannot see well may be uncertain and frightened of a strange environment.

● *What does the child say is the matter?*
Talking to children is an important way of understanding their experiences. Using play materials and drawing can establish rapport with the younger child and is a way of communicating with a child who finds it difficult to talk about unhappy events and feelings. It is important to convey interest in the child's point of view, but not to interrogate or ask why he or she has misbehaved. Conversation about family, friends, and school should be encouraged, and the interviewer should try to share in the child's feelings about their experiences.

● *What triggers the problem?*
It is often possible to identify events, perhaps something that is said or done, that sets off the behaviour problem. For example, the sight of a doctor may trigger off hysterical screaming; a parent's refusal to let the child do what he or she wants may set off a tantrum or an aggressive outburst. As well, some children behave worse with certain members of their family, or with certain ward staff, than with others.

● *How does the problem resolve?*
It is well known that the consequences of behaviour will affect the likelihood of it being repeated. For example, if children always get their own way by shouting and kicking, then they learn this behaviour is effective and will use it again. Because social attention is important to children, they will often behave inappropriately to gain adults' attention. Parents or nursing staff who only respond to children when they are being difficult, demanding, or naughty will find this type of behaviour increases over time.

One method of determining which factors may be maintaining the child's difficult behaviour is to keep an 'ABC' chart – Antecedents, Behaviour, and Consequences. Each time the problem behaviour occurs, the parent or nurse records what triggered the problem (antecedents), what the child does (behaviour), and what happens as a result (consequences):

Activity
Observe a child who is showing difficult and demanding behaviour on the ward and make an ABC chart during the course of the day. Identify the events that trigger the child's demands and observe both the staff and the parents' reactions to the child. Make sure you see the final outcome of any demand and decide whether the parent or child has had their own way. Try to decide what you think is maintaining the child's difficult behaviour.

Table 4.3 *ABC chart*

Antecedents	Behaviour	Consequences
Parent leaves ward.	Child screams.	Parent returns to cuddle child. Screaming stops.
Child sees toy being played with.	Snatches toy.	Other child gives in.
Child is refused a biscuit.	Kicks and screams.	Is given a biscuit. Kicking and screaming stops.

Assessing past experiences

What is family life like?
A child's experiences at home are a major factor in determining behaviour. Information about family relationships can be obtained by: interacting with the family; observing interactions between family members; asking questions about familial relationships.

How do the parents manage the child's behaviour?
The parents' style of management will significantly affect the child's behaviour. This can be determined both by interviewing and by observing interaction between the parents and child.

Parents may be very strict and punitive, or they may be inconsistent and erratic. Some frequently give way to the child and let him or her rule the house; others give way only after the child has persisted and started to become aggressive and disruptive. Beliefs in how a child should be disciplined vary markedly; and parents may say one thing but act differently.

What is the quality of the parent–child relationship?
A parent's emotional state can markedly affect the quality of their relationship with their child. A mother who is depressed may only respond to her child when goaded into action through naughty or unpleasant behaviour. A father who is anxious and worried may transfer his anxiety to the child. The parent may affect the child's development and behaviour by interfering excessively, not allowing the child to develop independence. A parent may be very rejecting, or they may be limited in the quality of relationship they can offer the child because of their own impoverished childhood. Emotional neglect and abuse is an important aspect of childhood behaviour problems.

Have there been any traumatic life events?
Unpleasant previous experiences in hospital, unhappy separations, or loss of a parent through death or divorce will all affect a child's emotions and behaviour. Studies of the occurrence of major life events demonstrate an association with changes in the level of behavioural and emotional problems in children (Berden *et al.*, 1990). It is not clear whether the effect of ongoing social and family variables outweighs the importance of significant life events, as children from disturbed or stressed families have higher levels of significant life events than other children.

The systematic formulation of the child's problem is the basis of the management and treatment plan. Barker (1988) describes a number of possible causative factors that need to be considered:

Predisposing factors: what pre-existing factors contributed to the development of the problem?
Precipitating factors: why did the problem appear at that particular time?
Perpetuating factors: what is maintaining the problem?
Protective factors: what are the child's and the family's strengths?

All of these factors should be considered in the context of environmental, temperamental, constitutional, and physical effects. Barker links these factors into a recording grid that can be updated as information is gained: see Table 4.4.

Table 4.4 *Formulation grid of contributing factors (Barker, 1988)*

	Constitu- tional	Tempera- mental	Physical	Environ- mental
Predisposing	–	Strong will	–	Parents' poor limit setting for the children
Participating	Had tonsillitis	–	–	Brother was going into parents' bed at night
Perpetuating	–	Argues with parents to get own way	–	Parents unable to make Sarah sleep in her own room
Protective	Well child	Bright extrovert girl	–	Close warm family

Exercise
A mother complains that her nine-year-old is out of control and never does anything she asks. What questions would you ask in order to define the problem more clearly and specifically?

Therapeutic approaches

As children's emotional and behavioural problems often have multiple causes, it may be necessary to use more than one form of treatment. The main therapeutic approaches include:

Family therapy   Counselling
Behaviour therapy   Hypnotherapy
Individual psychotherapy   Pharmacotherapy
Group therapy

The nurse's knowledge of the range of treatments available is important in understanding the role of other health professionals seeing the child, and also in enabling parents to find the help they require. In order to support families and provide a preventative service, nurses in the community can also develop a range of therapeutic skills. Counselling skills, group therapy and behaviour therapy all offer techniques that can be learned and used by nurses.

Family therapy

Here, the focus of therapy is the family system, with all of the family members participating. The way in which family members interrelate and communicate is the primary goal of intervention, rather than an individual member's mental or emotional state. It is expected that changes in the family system will lead to the resolution of the problem.

Behaviour therapy

This approach is based on learning theory and is an empirical approach to intervention. Precise targets for behaviour change are set, and the aim is to eliminate undesirable behaviours and to develop appropriate behaviours. Learning theory states that behaviour develops through conditioning experiences.

Classical conditioning occurs when events occur closely together in time, and the emotional effects produced by one event transfer to another event, for example, when a child learns to feel anxious about wasps after the mother panics on seeing one. Treatment involves desensitization whereby the child is taught to relax or enjoy playing with favourite toys, and the feared object is slowly reintroduced, eventually without evoking fear.

Operant conditioning is the modification of behaviour through the manipulation of the consequences of behaviour. The methods include positive reinforcement to increase desired behaviour, e.g. star charts for dry beds, and negative reinforcement and extinction to decrease undesired behaviour, e.g. ignoring tantrums. Parents can be taught to use these techniques effectively in order to improve their children's behaviour.

Individual psychotherapy

The basis of this approach is the development of the relationship between the therapist and the patient. There are many different types of psychotherapy, ranging from supportive psychotherapy, which aims to help the child cope better with the present situation, to psycho-analysis, which is a highly specialized long-term treatment that explores unconscious thoughts and fantasies.

Group therapy

Children or the parents of disturbed children may be treated in groups, the aim being to enable group members to help each other through their interaction and the modelling they provide for each other. The structure of the group can vary from a psychotherapeutic orientation to a problem-solving group aimed, for example, at helping parents to support each other in coping with their children's behaviour.

Counselling

This is often referred to as 'casework' and is the basis of many social workers' approach to treatment. It may, for example, involve facilitating environmental change by mobilizing community resources and support when families are in need of help. Some counsellors now work in schools with adolescents who are facing emotional crisis at home or with their peers.

Hypnotherapy

In hypnotherapy a state of deep relaxation is induced and awareness of events is heightened or decreased. Hypnotherapy can be used to help children gain access to unconscious thoughts and feelings, to promote physiological changes, gain control over anxiety-provoking events, achieve pain control, and improve self-esteem.

Pharmacotherapy

Medication has a role in the treatment of many childhood emotional disorders. Stimulants are used in the treatment of hyperactivity; anti-depressants for affective disorders; tranquillizers for anxiety states; and major tranquillizers for schizophrenia. Medication is not generally used for behavioural problems, although hypnotic drugs are used for sleep problems in young children, and anti-depressants are used in the treatment of diurnal enuresis.

Treatment of behaviour problems

Management of anti-social behaviour

Changes in the family environment and parental management are important features in changing children's anti-social behaviour. Behaviour therapy programmes that enable parents to establish clear and consistent controls over their children's behaviour have been proved to be effective. In observing and recording interchanges between parents and their anti-social children, Patterson (1982) found that coercive interactions were common, whereby family members would try to make others do as they wished by using aggression. One person would make a demand, which would be met with refusal, causing the first person to become more coercive. When aggressive or coercive behaviour successfully terminates the behaviour of the other person, the behaviour is reinforced and over time becomes worse. The cycle of interchange (Figure 4.2) can progress to violence and anger, accelerating to dangerous levels until the most violent person 'wins'.

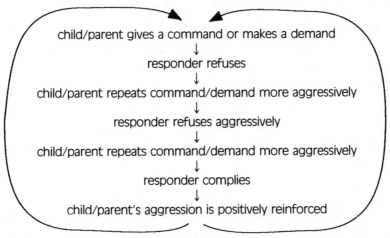

Figure 4.2 *Coercive behaviour in families of aggressive children*

Case study

Jake's mother had been observed by the nursery workers hitting him around the face and head. She always seemed stressed and anxious and had never talked to other parents or the nursery staff, and appeared unhappy and angry with Jake. The health visitor was asked to do some regular visiting and observed the aggressive interaction between Jake and his mother. He was destructive and demanding at home and the only way his mother could manage him was to threaten and smack him. The only way Jake could get his mother's attention was to be naughty or aggressive towards her and then she would shout at him.

Such families can be taught to establish clear behavioural goals by parents rewarding their children's social behaviour, and ignoring or extinguishing aggressive behaviour. Forehand and McMahon (1981) have described in detail a management approach to helping parents of aggressive and non-compliant children:

Phase 1

➤ The parent is taught to be a more effective reinforcer by increasing the number and range of reinforcers they offer the child, and by not using verbal behaviour that is associated with the child's non-compliance, that is, criticism, commands, and questions.

➤ The parent is trained to praise the child when he or she is being compliant or behaving well, that is, praise is dependent or contingent on the child's good behaviour. They learn the use of contingent attention to increase the child's good behaviour.

➤ The parent is taught to ignore minor inappropriate behaviours.

➤ The parent has a 10–15 minute period at home every day to practise the new behavioural skills and to focus on increasing the child's appropriate behaviour.

Phase 2

➤ The parent is trained to give direct, single commands. If the child complies, then the parent reinforces the child with praise and contingent attention.

➤ 'Time out' is used in response to the child's non-compliance. The child is warned they will have to sit on a chair in the corner of the room if they do not comply within five seconds. If the child doesn't comply, they are placed on the chair for three minutes and allowed to calm down for about 15 seconds. They are then asked again to comply.

Positive reinforcement

Some children who show particularly difficult behaviour need to receive recognition of their good behaviour in order to make it seem important and worth trying to do. Privileges that can be earned in a systematic way, or using a wall chart with stickers or stars to indicate that the child has behaved well can help a child feel successful, thus building self-esteem (Herbert, 1987).

Any type of chart or token given for good behaviour should be carefully managed and understood by the ward team and the parents. Everyone, including the child, must know clearly what the child must do to 'earn' a sticker. The child should be carefully monitored so that stickers are given appropriately, and not because no-one noticed what happened over the past hour! When the stickers are given, they should be accompanied by praise and recognition of how good he or she has been.

The social reward of being given the sticker is more important than the sticker itself: if the sticker is given by someone who does not know

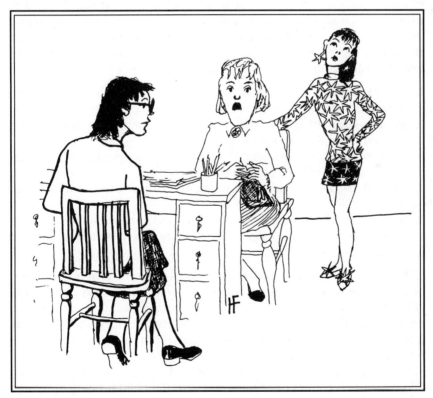

I am so pleased. Your star reward system has completely cured Marlene's obsession.

the child, or who sees it as just another chore, the value of the chart is easily lost, and the child feels it is no longer worth trying. This applies to all situations in which star charts are used for behaviour problems, whether at home, school, or in hospital, and also for all types of behaviour problems, whether for dry beds, or finishing a plate of food.

Exercise
Write out what you might say when describing the use of a star chart to a mother to help her child stop bed wetting. What is the most important element in using the chart? (Suggested answers at end of book.)

Teaching alternative behaviour

Many aggressive children have a limited range of reactions to conflicts with adults and other children: they automatically threaten, swear, or use physical aggression. Such children may need help in trying to think of other ways to respond, and to anticipate the outcomes of other strategies. Spivak *et al.* (1976) have developed a treatment programme that helps aggressive children to solve their social problems more effectively by focusing on their thought processes. This includes teaching the children five main processes.

1. **Alternative solution thinking**: the child is encouraged to generate different solutions to interpersonal conflicts.
2. **Means–end thinking**: the child is taught to understand the steps needed to attain a solution.
3. **Consequential thinking**: the child learns to identify what might be the results of each solution.
4. **Causal thinking**: the child understands how one event leads to another.
5. **Sensitivity to interpersonal problems**: the child is taught to become aware of problems and to identify potential difficulties with others.

Children need feedback about their good behaviour. When the child is behaving well, it is important for the nurse or parents to sit with the child for a few minutes and make comments that praise and demonstrate genuine interest. It is also helpful for nurses to take some time to play with or talk to the child regularly so there is a chance for a relationship to develop.

Parents and nurses need to decide which behaviours can be ignored and which behaviours need to be stopped. If a child is being noisy and restless they can be ignored, but if he or she starts to interfere with other children or become disruptive, then intervention is necessary. If the behaviour cannot be ignored, the child must know clearly what is not permitted; there should be consistent and clear expectations so the child knows what will happen if they step over the mark. If a time-out approach is used, the child must have the opportunity to come back and try again in order to learn appropriate behaviour.

Exercise

A six-year-old boy is hitting others in the play-room on the ward in order to get his own way. His mother is present but is not intervening. What could you do? (Suggested answers at end of book.)

Management of hyperactivity and attention deficit disorder

Hyperactive children require continual supervision and attention. When left unoccupied and unsupervised they often get into mischief, climbing on furniture, touching and fiddling with equipment on the ward, rushing around in a dangerous and disruptive manner, breaking objects, or being accidentally destructive.

These children respond best to a structured routine in safe surroundings, where they are not continually being reprimanded but gain positive feedback about their behaviour. They need planned, structured activities that keep them busy. Parents often require help and support in managing these children. Behaviour management is useful, as well as advice about organization and supervision in the home. Kendall and Braswell (1985) have used a cognitive behavioural method to teach self control to impulsive and hyperactive children. Children are taught to think out loud initially so that their thought processes become apparent and structured. The self-instructional training has five steps.

1. Problem definition: learning to clarify and understand the requirements of the task.
2. Problem approach: learning to plan a general strategy.
3. Focusing attention.
4. Selecting an answer.
5. Self-reinforcing for correct performance.

Hyperactivity is one of the few behavioural problems that respond to medication. This choice of treatment method accentuates the importance of having an accurate assessment and diagnosis of the condition. The confusion that often occurs between the diagnosis of conduct disordered and hyperactive or attention deficit disordered children can lead to inappropriate treatment methods being used and being ineffective.

Dietary management of hyperactivity has become an accepted form of treatment recently for a small number of children. In a rigorous study, Egger *et al.* (1985) put 76 hyperactive children on to an oligoantigenic (few foods) diet for four weeks. Foods were reintroduced in a systematic and gradual manner over several weeks, and parents recorded any change in their child's behaviour during that time. Twenty-eight children who appeared to react to certain foods were placed back on to the oligoantigenic diet, and capsules that possibly contained the identified food given to the child to eat. Neither the parents nor the researchers knew if the capsules contained the suspect food.

All of the families demonstrated that their children's behaviour was better while taking the placebo, that is capsules that did not contain provocative foods. The foods most commonly implicated in producing a behavioural effect were benzoic acid and tartrazine together, but 46 other provocative foods were identified. The results indicate that combinations of many different foods can adversely affect some children's behaviour, and the attention now being paid to additives in children's food has some bearing in research findings.

Management of behaviour problems in young children

Difficulties with sleeping, eating, and toileting can concern parents as well as being a problem on the ward. Such problems may have started with a medical problem, but when they continue beyond the resolution of the organic problems they can be considered to be maintained by psycho-social factors. The child may have learned a particular way of behaving, which may be exacerbated by the parents' response to the problem. In other instances, the problem is due to inappropriate parental management techniques, which were present from the beginning.

There are some basic styles of management that apply to most behavioural problems, but their effectiveness lies in a good quality relationship between parent and child. With a child who feels rejected or who has been abused, no amount of management advice will succeed until the basic difficulty in the parenting relationship has been resolved.

Behavioural techniques can be applied to many different problems of early childhood, and have been shown to be particularly effective with sleep problems (Richman, *et al.*, 1985). The techniques commonly used are the following.

(i) Gradual behaviour change

Limits to the child's behaviour are introduced gradually so the child has a chance to learn what is expected without being confronted by a big change all at once. A child who will not settle to sleep without being cuddled can be taught to endure separation by gradually reducing contact over the course of several nights, so the child does not become distressed (Douglas and Richman, 1984). A child with a poor appetite can gradually be offered small amounts of food that are manageable, rather than a large plate of food. The aim is to teach the child to finish the food and to then feel successful at having achieved their goal. Once the child can reliably eat a small portion, the amount of food can gradually be increased (Douglas, 1991). A child can be toilet trained by being encouraged to sit on the potty for short periods of time. They are unlikely to perform, but encouraging them to sit for longer and longer, and then introducing the idea of urinating or defecating into the potty will help to make the child aware of what is required.

(ii) Setting conditions for behaviour change

Children with behaviour problems have often come to recognize the wrong cues for their behaviour. For example, children who will not go to bed until very late may associate bedtime with seeing their parents going to bed. If a simple, finite bedtime routine is established, they can learn rapidly what is expected (Douglas and Richman, 1984). Children who only eat food on the run or throughout the day may need to learn to associate food with mealtimes at the table. If parents only offer food at set times, and only while the child sits at the table, the child will rapidly learn more appropriate eating patterns (Richman, 1988).

(iii) Increasing good behaviour

Praising children and giving them positive attention is a powerful way of increasing desired behaviour. Star charts, tokens that can be exchanged for privileges, outings, or presents are all ways of giving the child feedback about their success. They offer a way of increasing the child's motivation to change quickly, until the positive comments from the parent are sufficient to maintain the new behaviour. Reinforcers can be used for many different types of behaviour change, for example, staying in bed all night, trying a new food, using the potty, or having a dry bed.

(iv) Eliminating inappropriate behaviour

Parents and nursing staff can help young children behave more appropriately by ignoring their demanding and unco-operative behaviour and providing attention and praise when they behave well. Crying at night or faddiness about foods will often resolve when ignored.

Exercise

A mother complains that her two-year-old wakes five times a night and needs a bottle and a cuddle before he falls asleep again. What techniques could help the mother to teach her child to sleep through the night? (Suggested answers at end of book.)

Management of enuresis and encopresis

Enuresis

Once any physical causes have been excluded, then a conditioning treatment approach is often used. For nocturnal enuresis a bell-and-pad or night alarm can be used. This is a pad that is placed on the child's bed, and when the child urinates an alarm is activated that wakes the child. The child should then be sent to the toilet to urinate completely, the bed remade, and the alarm reset. In one study, 84% of 113 children improved but 40 relapsed. Of the 31 who were re-treated, 16 remained dry, giving a long-term success rate of 63% (Dische *et al.*, 1983).

Daytime wetting can be treated in the same way with a portable pants alarm, which was found to be effective in two-thirds of children. There appeared to be no difference in the effect between having a contingent alarm that was activated by urine, or a non-contingent alarm that went off intermittently and reminded the child to go to the toilet (Halliday *et al.*, 1987).

Encopresis

Treatment approaches should be linked to the assessment of the type of encopresis shown by the child. Behavioural methods of management are often used, sometimes in conjunction with laxatives and stool-softening agents if retention is a feature. Once the constipation is treated, providing a structured and reinforcing programme for the child with star charts and incentives can enable the child to learn to pass motions appropriately.

Case study

Tim had never passed a motion in the toilet and at the age of four years had to have a nappy on just to pass a motion. He was severely constipated, often stained his pants and had tried a range of medication. He refused to sit on the toilet and his mother was desperate for help as she kept losing her temper with him. A simple reinforcement programme was started with mother offering Tim a surprise from a bag of small presents if he would just sit on the toilet. Within a day, Tim's curiosity had won and he agreed to sit on the toilet briefly in order to find out what the surprise present was. Over the course of the next week he had been encouraged to sit on the toilet for up to 10 minutes four times a day in order to receive a small surprise. The next stage was to offer a surprise if he was able to pass a motion in the toilet. This he was able to do successfully with the help of medication initially. Both Tim and his mother were delighted with the progress and Tim was very proud that he was able to use the toilet.

If the retention is due to emotional problems based in the family relationships, then a family therapy approach may be necessary.

If the encopresis is non-retentive and continuous, the child may need an intensive period of learning what to do and where to do it. Frequent opportunities to sit on the toilet or the potty need to be scheduled into the day, or at times that the child is likely to wet or soil themselves, so that he or she has a higher chance of performing in the right place (Hersov, 1985).

If the encopresis is discontinuous, then family therapy is often needed to address the parent–child conflict, and to establish more appropriate expectations and patterns of behaviour control in the family (Barker, 1988).

Management of adolescent behaviour problems

Drug and substance abuse

Adolescent drug abuse is very difficult to treat, particularly if motivation to change is minimal. Many may not stop until they have a significant experience that makes them see drugs in a different light. While there are drug treatment centres where adolescents can receive therapy while stopping, problems of relapse after discharge are significant. Self-help organisations like Alcoholics Anonymous or Narcotics Anonymous may also be helpful, but these are based on the adolescent accepting the fact of addiction and wanting to take control of their life again. A community-based approach to prevention and education may be more significant, although it is difficult to assess the impact and deterrent value of public health advertisements on drug abuse and smoking.

Treatment of emotional problems

Management of fears and phobias

Nurses frequently encounter fears and phobias related to hospitals and medical procedures on the ward, and often have a central role in helping the child overcome these fears. Systematic desensitization is the most common form of treatment for fears and phobias. This may occur in the child's imagination while feeling relaxed, or may occur in reality (Graziano *et al.*, 1979).

School refusal is a common problem and management of it involves an accurate assessment of the reason for the problem, and often requires family therapy. The family may need help to enable the child to separate from home successfully. Co-operation between home and school is important in order to enable teachers to understand the problem. The child's return to school needs to be carefully planned to reduce the level of tension as much as possible, and the child should be fully involved in the planning and be aware of the necessity of returning to school. Sometimes a professional, for example, an educational welfare officer, social worker or school nurse may need to take the child to school for a few days in order to overcome the child's high resistance, which the parents cannot handle. It is important that the child does not have the experience of staying at home to reduce their anxiety once they have returned to school (Barker, 1988). Blagg and Yule (1984) describe a treatment approach with several flexible elements:

- Detailed clarification of the child's problem.
- Realistic discussion of child, parental, and teacher worries.
- Contingency plans to ensure maintenance once the child has returned to school.
- An enforced return to school, under escort if necessary.
- Follow-up contact until the child is attending full time for six weeks.

Twenty-eight out of thirty children treated using this approach returned rapidly to school, while a comparison group treated in a hospital inpatient unit did less well. Another group treated by home teaching and outpatient psychotherapy did very poorly.

Management of obsessional thoughts and compulsive rituals

Many children show minor forms of obsessional and ritualistic behaviour, like avoiding stepping on the cracks in the pavement, but sometimes the compulsions become disruptive to normal life. These thoughts and actions are usually carried out to ward off an anticipated, imaginary, unpleasant event. Many children worry that something might happen to them or to their parents if they do not carry out these rituals or if they think the thoughts. Behavioural treatment is usually by response prevention. By stopping the child from repeating the thoughts or actions, they are forced to realize that nothing terrible happens if they do not complete them. This relieves the anxiety, and the child can then stop the behaviour (Stanley, 1980).

Management of psychosomatic disorders

Feelings of stress, anxiety, and worry can give rise to a range of physical symptoms, which is often the way the child expresses that something is wrong. They may have bottled up their feelings and have no other way of demonstrating their worries. Management of psychosomatic disorders should not focus only on the physical symptoms, but attempt to understand the reason for the problem. Parents may be so worried about the child's physical symptoms that they exacerbate the problem rather than ameliorate it. In severe cases, the child may have several operations in order to identify the cause of a pain which in reality has no physical basis. Nurses should be aware that parents may ask for several different opinions, or take the child around to many different hospitals.

Parents' complaints should always be treated with respect and understanding. The child may appear to be attention-demanding and manipulative, but in fact they are expressing a painful emotional problem in the only way they know. Sometimes the problems are rooted in the family, and the distortion in family relationships is the basis of the difficulties being shown by the child. If this is the case, they need specialist help from a psychiatrist or psychologist, who can work with the family in therapy.

Psychosomatic complaints should not be challenged or ignored, but recognized as a cry for help. The nurse should also be aware of the distinction between psychosomatic behaviour in children, and Munchausen (by proxy) syndrome in the parents, who artificially create symptoms in their children to gain medical treatment.

Management of depression in children

Treatment of depression involves identifying the causal factors for the depression and providing help around those issues. Problems within family relationships may need to be approached through family therapy; physical and sexual abuse or emotional neglect may need to be managed through removal of the child from the family to a place of safety; problems at school may need to be addressed with teachers, with individual help being offered to the child. In severe cases, anti-depressant medication may be necessary. If a child is expressing suicidal thoughts, then admission to hospital may be necessary for safety and psychiatric treatment.

Nurses' ability to listen to children and to help them to talk about what is worrying them may be a vital part of treatment; children may reveal worries and upsets they have never been able to express before. Their concerns need to be understood with sympathy and constructive aid. They often need the chance or the opportunity to learn how to express their feelings.

Exercise

A ten-year-old girl is admitted for investigation of nausea and abdominal pain. She seems lively and happy when her mother is not on the ward. Devise an observational plan for staff on the ward in order to watch her reactions in different situations and with different people present. Think about how you would code her behaviour and the kind of chart you could use for this. (Suggested answers at end of book.)

Management of mental illness

Childhood schizophrenia

Families with a schizophrenic child require long-term support and help in understanding the disorder. Anti-psychotic drugs can be used, but the long-term use of drugs can lead to serious side-effects and so doses need to be kept low. This is a very serious disorder with poor outcome. The earlier the onset of symptoms the more damage is likely to occur to the development of the child's personality and psychological growth. Sudden onset has been associated with better prognosis, and sometimes complete recovery (Barker, 1988).

Disintegrative psychoses

Some medication can be used to alleviate some of the symptoms, but the progressive disorders may be fatal and devastating to the child's family. The level of brain damage that has occurred will severely affect the child's functioning, and may cause severe mental retardation. The families need long-term support, and help in the community to cope with caring for the child (Barker, 1988).

The community nurse in particular may be involved in supporting the family with a psychotic child. The stress and family management issues that a mentally ill child can create involve the community services in long-term care.

Summary

Children's behavioural and emotional problems may be linked to their special needs, illness or family life experiences. Dealing with these issues is often highly stressful for nurses, and also for families. This chapter has described the different types of emotional and behavioural problems that nurses will encounter and provides an outline of the assessment and interviewing skills that nurses can use.

Assessment and interviewing skills are an essential part of the nurse's role. Being aware of the need for reliable information, but also how to elicit thoughts and feelings about the child's and the family's problems create the basis for a treatment and intervention plan. A systematic and sensitive assessment approach will help prevent the nurse from making inappropriate judgements or false assumptions. The use of behavioural charts can be valuable not only for parents, but also to understand interactions with difficult children on the ward and at home.

A range of treatment methods are described, not all of which a nurse will use, but which illustrate the possible types of treatment available. Nurses can utilize many components of these treatments in their daily management of children on the ward and also while advising parents at home.

More detailed descriptions of behaviour management techniques are given as these are methods that nurses can incorporate into their repertoire of skills. Management of aggression, sleep, eating and toilet problems in young children are often presented as particular areas of concern by parents. Children who show symptoms of anxiety or depression may develop psychosomatic symptoms or require help to overcome their fears and worries.

Further reading

Barker, P. (1988). *Basic Child Psychiatry 5th ed.* Blackwell Scientific Publications, Oxford.
A readable overview of the main psychiatric problems shown by children and an introduction to different types of treatment for these disorders.

Douglas, J. (1989). *Behaviour Problems in Young Children.* Tavistock/Routledge London.
Provides a comprehensive and practical introduction for nursing and medical staff to the management of the common behaviour problems of young children that concern parents.

SECTION TWO
Caring for sick children

5 Caring for sick children in the community

The psychological effects of chronic disease

Children with chronic disease may be more vulnerable to problems in their emotional and behavioural development, particularly those who have suffered damage to their central nervous system, for example, epilepsy, or have a physical disability such as cerebral palsy. Most children with chronic illness, however, adjust to the stresses and demands of their condition, for instance only about one-fifth of children with chronic renal failure have been found to show emotional problems (Garralda *et al.*, 1988). Younger children appear to be more affected in their school work and level of attainment at school (Allen and Zigler, 1986), while older children are affected more in their social adjustment and ability to make friends (Ungerer *et al.*, 1988).

The effect of having a chronically ill child in the family is unpredictable, and will often vary. A child's response to their illness is, in turn, affected by the family's reaction to the problems. Those with a chronically ill child experience similar problems to any other family – marital difficulties, divorce, distress, and psychopathology – but this should not be interpreted as a reaction to the stress of having a chronically ill child so much as a reflection of the way the family copes with problems in general. The methods of coping that family members use will help to determine whether they manage the stress and adapt to it or become incapacitated by it. Perrin and MacLean (1988) concluded that divorce is no higher among parents of chronically ill children than among the general population.

How the family copes

There has been a considerable change in the approach to conceptualizing the impact of chronic disease on children and their families in recent years. The traditional deficit-centered model is gradually being replaced by models that take into account coping resources and individual competence. Instead of an emphasis on psychopathology in families, there is a growing understanding of how families cope with crises; they are viewed as ordinary people coping with exceptional circumstances (Eiser, 1990). Unfortunately, many studies are still based on the view that chronic disease has a negative psychological impact. This approach has few implications for prevention and intervention with families, while an emphasis on how children and families can learn appropriate coping strategies creates a more positive and therapeutic orientation (Fehrenbach and Peterson, 1989).

Varni and Wallander (1988) have proposed a model to analyse the impact of chronic illness in families. They propose reciprocal interaction between three types of variables:

1. Intrapersonal factors, including the severity of the handicap, functional independence, and personality factors like the temperament and coping style of the child.
2. Interpersonal factors, including the temperament and coping style of the mother.
3. Socio-ecological factors, including marital and family functioning, socio-economic status, family size, and service utilization.

They suggest that families with chronically ill children are more at risk of maladjustment because of the increased number of stressful situations requiring a solution or decision for appropriate action.

Exercise
Make a list of the potential problematic situations faced, and decisions that need to be made, by the family of a ten-year-old child with chronic asthma, and by the family of a one-year-old child with leukaemia. (Suggested answers at end of book).

The family management style

Given the fluctuating and changing nature of many children's chronic conditions, the community health practitioner should focus on understanding the processes of managing the child's illness in the family, and be alert to the interactions between family members and how this affects their ability to cope.

The 'family management style' is an active and interactive process that has been described by Knafl and Deatrick (1990), who have outlined a comprehensive assessment schedule for families with a diabetic child; this could be used equally well with other chronic illnesses. There are three main components.

1. *Assessment of the social and cultural attitudes of the family.* Every family has values and beliefs that will affect how they react and cope with illness in their child.

2. *Assessment of how each member feels.* Each person in the family has their own way of identifying the important aspects of the illness and its effect on family life. Each has different feelings about the illness, which will mean different things to each person.

3. *Assessment of how each member of the family copes.* This is closely bound up with their definition of the situation. Adjustments may or may not be made by each member of the family, and by the family as a whole, to accommodate the illness.

Exercise

Milos is a four-year-old boy who has cystic fibrosis. He has an elder brother aged ten and a sister aged seven. He attends nursery four mornings a week. While reading the next sections, consider how you might assess the differing impact on his mother (a housewife) and father (a travelling salesman) of his daily care routine.

Assessment of social and cultural attitudes

Each family has a culturally defined meaning of illness that permits the ill child to receive special care and attention and to adopt a special role (Anderson, 1986). Being ill may mean the child is absolved of responsibility for tasks and jobs in the home, or they may get special foods and gifts; the child may also not be punished for difficult behaviour or naughtiness. Such attitudes could conflict with that of health care professionals, who tend to feel that chronically ill children should lead as independent and normal a life as possible. If the conflict in attitudes is not noticed or discussed, the family is likely to find nursing support unhelpful, and may undermine it in some way.

In some families, the economic considerations of caring for the ill child are immense. Sometimes, a parent may have to give up work in order to be at home with the child. In others, the costs of transport to hospital and clinic appointments adds additional stress to an over-stretched family budget.

Chronic illness can arouse a political awareness in some families, who will start to fight for resources for their child, or for children with the particular illness, through joining or creating pressure groups, lobbying for resources, or by publicity. The nurse is a resource provider, but also has a role in improving services and service delivery.

In trying to understand their child's illness, some families find support and meaning from their religious faith. They may see the illness as a test of their faith and commitment, and are therefore able to draw on inner reserves in order to cope. In other families, a fatalistic attitude to the course of the illness may be adopted. Such parents may not fight for the needs of their child, but passively accept that this is how things are. Some parents may see the illness as a judgement on them for sins of the past, and feel guilty or blamed for the illness.

Social and ethnic attitudes will help to determine who cares for the child at home. Mothers usually take on most of the caring role, but the level of sharing of daily tasks and responsibility will be determined in part by the cultural expectations in the family. The sex of the ill child may also determine the type of care and treatment they receive.

Assessment of how each family member feels

Each person in the family has a view about how the child's illness is affecting them, how it has changed their life, and what it means to them in their daily life. This information can help the health professional to build up a picture of what meaning the illness has in the family, what are the stresses and strains, and how the illness has changed emotional relationships. Family members may differ in their perception of the seriousness of the illness, how they should cope with it, and how they should treat the ill child (Gallo, 1990).

Medical and nursing contact is mostly with the child's mother which, because it presents only one perspective, can be unreliable in terms of what is happening in the family. The mother may be concerned about the effect of the ill child's treatment regime on the family diet, the time required to administer medication or treatment, or the additional 'washing and cleaning that is necessary. To her, the illness creates more work and responsibility (Gibson, 1988).

Case study

Mrs Simon was feeling over-stressed by looking after her five-year-old son, who had cerebral palsy. She was not sharing the responsibility of his care with her husband, and found it difficult to allow him to take any independent action in relation to John's illness. She frequently complained that her husband didn't help out and that she had to make all the decisions, but in reality she was unable to let her husband join in. Mrs Simon complained of feeling depressed and exhausted, but continually worried about John's welfare. She had become rigid about the daily routine of exercises and stimulation, and found that every minute of the day was taken up with some form of special care for John. She felt her life was totally devoted to him, and that there was no one who could carry out all the necessary tasks as well as she could. She had refused all offers of respite care and help in the home.

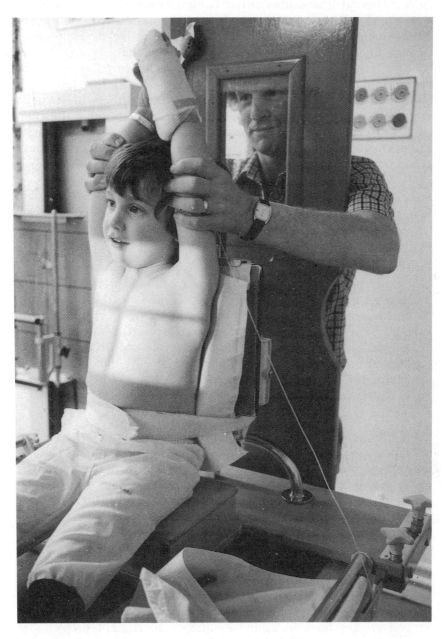

The father may have a very different perspective. He may have a different period of adjustment to his child's chronic illness, often taking longer to absorb the impact of the illness because of a reduced level of contact with the child, and may feel and show his feelings differently. He may find that his daily routine is not affected greatly, except that family activities at weekends or holiday times are curtailed or altered by the child's condition. Other fathers take an active role in helping at home and carrying responsibility for the child. Fathers may forego promotion or job changes in order to be near the hospital the child visits, or to keep shorter working hours in order to help out at home. Parents might not acknowledge the differences in each other's feelings or attitudes, and this can create tension between them.

Case study

Mrs Trent reported feeling very lonely since the birth of her little girl with spina bifida. She felt as if she was alone in coping with the baby. She had desperately wanted to share her feelings and worries with her husband, but they could never talk about Claire. She began to feel resentful towards her husband, and thought he didn't care about her or Claire. In fact, Mr Trent had avoided talking about Claire because he couldn't bear to see his wife cry. He worried continually about Claire, but couldn't see how he could make the situation any better. He felt completely helpless and hopeless, but didn't want to burden his wife with his feelings.

Ill children often have individual concerns that centre on the feelings the illness creates in them. They may be uncomfortable or in pain, or they may be worried about symptoms and the course of the illness. The restrictions imposed by their illness may create feelings of frustration and anger. Dietary restrictions, taking unpleasant medicine, or having regular injections may all be resented. They may feel upset that they have restricted activities at school, or that their schooling is interrupted by hospital visits. They may resent the fact that their illness makes them different from other children, and may take great efforts to conceal the fact that they are ill – or, they may not mind everyone knowing, and just treat their condition as part of life.

The effects on siblings' emotional development can also be significant. Several studies have identified emotional adjustment problems in siblings (Lavigne and Ryan, 1979; Cairns *et al.*, 1979) but other studies have found no significant difference in adjustment levels between siblings of well and chronically ill children (Gath, 1972; Breslau *et al.*, 1981). Siblings sometimes take on high levels of responsibility and care

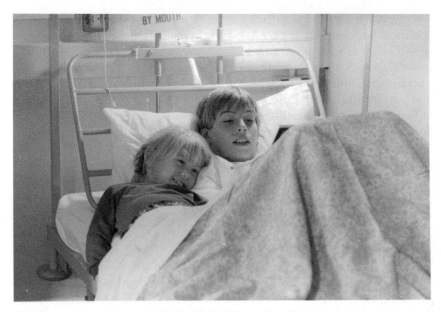

© Mike Hardy and Action for Sick Children. Reproduced by permission.

of their brother or sister; they may even become 'pseudo parents' and take on too much responsibility for their age, leading to feelings of resentment. Well siblings, especially females, may be expected to take on increased responsibilities in the house, and carry out child-care tasks and parent support while the expectations of the ill child are drastically reduced.

A sibling's response to growing up with a child with chronic illness varies according to the sibling's age, gender, developmental level, birth order, spacing, and type of illness (Brett, 1988). A young sibling may worry that he or she may catch or develop the same illness as their brother or sister (Thibodeau, 1988). A sense of guilt may develop if they feel they have caused the illness, or wished it on their sibling in a fit of temper. They may be upset by being separated from their parents when the ill child goes to hospital, and they may feel jealous and angry. The junior-aged child may get upset about small events, and feel resentful that their ill sibling gets so much attention.

The junior-age group can be self-centred and interested only in their own friendships and activities. They can feel irritated that their sibling's illness gets in the way of their activities. Occasionally they may feel guilty about their selfishness, but underlying this is a resentment that having a chronically ill brother or sister makes them different from other children.

Some siblings feel guilty that they are well; their concern for their ill sibling will be great, and they empathize strongly with their sibling's feelings. Some children may have very inaccurate or immature views about what is wrong with their ill sibling, which may frighten them.

Adolescents may fluctuate between wanting to help at home and carry responsibility for their ill sibling, and wanting to break away from the family and lead independent lives. They may request detailed information about the illness, and also worry about the implications for themselves and their own children.

Nurses should be aware of the impact of the child's illness on different members of the family, and make a particular effort to include all members' views in the initial assessment of the family functioning. The parents also need to realize the varying effect that the illness has, and be aware of the needs of the siblings.

Management of the ill child

One focus of the family will be the accommodation to the child's medical state and treatment requirements, so the assessment of the family's coping methods should include details of that process. Who gives the medication, does the exercises, checks the blood, carries out tests at home, takes the child to appointments or treatment? Is it one person, shared, systematic, or erratic? Are the necessary functions for maintaining the child at home being carried out effectively? If not, what is going wrong, and how can the family members negotiate and agree on a plan of action?

Areas of responsibility may need to be defined, or a transfer of responsibility may need to be negotiated. Gibson (1988) provided questionnaires to 56 parents of children with cystic fibrosis, and found that all experienced a degree of illness-related stress. They noted problems with carrying out the prescribed treatment regimens, in particular the chest physiotherapy, which was time consuming. They reported difficulties in scheduling time for the other members of the family, and also difficulty in finding someone to look after the child so the family could have some respite from care.

Management of the family

If the focus is the family system, then it is important to identify how relationships and roles in the family are affected. Minuchin *et al.* (1978) have developed a comprehensive model of family functioning to explain the effect of illness on the family. This model is derived from studies of children with diabetes, asthma, and anorexia nervosa. They propose that there is a common pattern of family interaction, irrespective of the particular illness. Minuchin developed the term 'psychosomatic family' to describe the maladaptive interactions that are characterized by:

- over-protectiveness, i.e., morbid concern for each other;
- enmeshment, i.e., the lack of generation boundaries between parents and children;
- rigidity, i.e., the inability to adapt to the child's developing needs;
- lack of conflict resolution, i.e., the avoidance of disagreements and the failure to resolve problems.

Such families frequently show ineffective parental control and supervision; a child who is overdependent or out of control; a child and one parent in opposition to the other parent; the family resistant to change, as the maladaptive interactions prevent the emergence of potentially more harmful conflicts within the family system.

But many families do make successful adaptations to the needs of the chronically ill child. Ritchie (1981) found that families with an epileptic member were more efficient at decision-making tasks than control families, demonstrating the possible beneficial effects of adaptation to stress. Successful adaptation depends on appropriate cognitive assessment of the problems, and the use of effective behavioural responses or coping strategies. One study found that many parents of children with osteogenesis imperfecta made a particular effort to create a normal family life by going out together as a couple, or by planning family outings and activities (Deatrick *et al.*, 1988).

The fact that families can alter and adapt to new circumstances demonstrates their flexibility. Underlying strengths are often revealed, and some parents may even feel they have benefited as they have grown closer in their relationship, and have had to evaluate the meaning of their own lives in a less selfish and self-centred way. They may have taken time to think about their own priorities, and consequently feel happier about the reasons for their actions. Siblings may be closer or may have developed a more altruistic, caring approach to relationships with others. They may be more mature and more tolerant, and so have better social skills with which to cope with the world outside the family (Brett, 1988).

Whether families are co-ordinated and co-operative in their management style, or conflictual and erratic may have nothing to do with the child's illness. All families experience some marital and parent–child conflicts; problems in discipline and child management occur universally. How the family copes with these normal problems will therefore affect how they cope with the additional stresses created by an ill child which may exacerbate and highlight the underlying conflicts and disagreements. Families do break up with the stress of looking after a chronically ill child, but it may be that the problems pre-existed the diagnosis of the illness.

Management of the social system

If the focus is the social system, then parents will be considering the effects of the child's illness on the world outside the home. They may be occupied with arranging special tuition or extra help for their child. They may need to make decisions about who should be told about the illness and what should they be told; how the illness will be managed at school and what special schooling requirements will be needed by the child; which professionals need to be involved in order to gain services, what services are available, and what do they need. The family also needs to decide who is going to carry out these actions. At times they may be shared, while at other times one person may elect to do the required task.

The family may use social support outside the family. or they may try to cope on their own. They may feel they do not want to burden others with their problems, or that no one else can really understand or help them. They may reject and denigrate support from professionals. Other families find the social support they receive from friends, relatives, and professionals an important part of being able to cope.

In a case study of a diabetic eight-year-old and her family, Deatrick and Knafl (1990) have presented an analysis of the family management behaviours (see Table 5.1). It may be helpful for the nurse to draw up a similar daily, weekly, or monthly assessment chart for each family in their care in order to determine the effects on the family and to pinpoint any areas of deficit.

A chart like this can help the nurse to assess a range of family behaviours. The nurse can then help the family to examine what they are doing, who is doing it, and the goals of their activities. After the assessment, the family members may wish to re-negotiate their roles with each other, or with the health and community support team. A common area of concern as the child grows is the developmental progression in the child's need for independence and control over their own condition. It is necessary to re-negotiate who implements the care so the responsibility shifts from the parent to the child.

This type of assessment can also guide the nurse in understanding the effects of hospitalization on chronically ill children and the additional stress it can provoke. The stress generated by repeated hospital admissions include parents worrying about the maintenance of care procedures; the idiosyncratic procedures and routines established at home; worry about the child's complex and personal ways of carrying out the activities of daily life; the maintenance of family routines.

The nurse must be aware of not making assumptions about a family's reaction to a child's chronic illness, e.g., that a family has full information about the child's condition and treatment; that a standard

Table 5.1 *Analysis of family management behaviours (Deatrick and Knafl, 1990)*

Target behaviour	Goal	Focus	Implementor
Test child's blood	Prevent low blood sugar	Child's illness	Mother
Tell school about disease	Image of child	Social system	Mother
Plan meals out	1. Normal family activities	Family system	Mother
	2. Maintain treatment	Child's illness	Mother & Father
Parents go out	Normal marital activities	Family system	Father
Attend support group	Information	Social system	Mother & Father

Exercise

Fill in the following family management plan for a family with a ten-year-old boy with cystic fibrosis.

Target behaviour	Goal	Focus	Implementor
?	Prevent chest congestion	Child's illness	?
?	Normal marital relationship	?	?
Ask for school work to be brought home	?	?	?
Family go swimming	?	?	Sibling
Hospital visit	?	?	?

(Answers at end of book.)

management approach is appropriate for all families with a chronically ill child; or that all families would benefit from joining a parent support group. The nurse should attempt to identify these assumptions and test them out empirically. There is also a specificity–generality issue and the nurse should be aware of the specific needs of families with, for example, a child with diabetes as distinct from a family with a child with cystic fibrosis.

Styles of coping in families

Each family will develop different coping strategies, some of which are successful and some of which are not. Lists of successful coping methods have been compiled by researchers, and combine to form six main strategies (Brett, 1988).

Social support

Many families cope by using social support, sharing the burden of chronic illness with friends, relatives, and professionals. Gibson (1988) found that parents of children with cystic fibrosis specified first the spouse or family as being the most supportive; second, the multi-disciplinary team in the cystic fibrosis clinic; and third, the Cystic Fibrosis Foundation, where they could meet other parents in the same situation. Self-help groups are an effective source of support for some parents, the ill child and well siblings. Nurses can facilitate the development of, or the contact with, self-help groups, and can also be a resource of information about possible support and resources from other professionals and agencies.

Normalization

Parents try to minimize the differences between children in the family, and most try to integrate the ill child into normal society and life as much as possible. Normalization can be an effective coping strategy as it minimizes the impact of the illness by maximizing the child's abilities, and also reduces the parents' level of anxiety and provides a sense of hope. The nurse can help by providing accurate and age appropriate information and support to the children about the illness and the feelings it produces. The parents can also be helped by examining and working through their own reactions and attitudes to illness in the family.

Mastery

Parents attempt to master the specific demands imposed by the illness, which will tend to decrease anxiety and increase levels of confidence and a sense of control. When individuals perceive that their ability to cope is greater than the demands confronting them, they feel a sense of personal control that is rewarding and positive. Mastery occurs through seeking out information about the disorder and learning how to manage and comply with the treatment requirements. Practical help may be sought from professionals or outside agencies like support groups and societies in order to permit the family to be independent and to cope with each new problem as it arises. Parents have a high and continuing need for information when they are coping with daily fluctuations in the child's health.

Being a support and a resource for advice and information can be a critical role for the nurse in alleviating stress in families. The nurse may also be required to help balance the care needs of the child with the parents' needs for occasional respite, and the siblings' needs for individual attention.

Understanding

Parents often try to attribute meaning to the experience of illness. They need to understand why it has happened to their child, and to them. This can lead to a transformation in their own beliefs and values: instead of feeling angry about the condition, it is accepted and integrated into their view of their own lives. The re-definition of personal beliefs is a slow and painful process, and families may need a long period of support by health professionals.

Communication

Families who communicate openly and in which each person can express their feelings or request information freely without fear of recrimination, secrecy or lies tend to cope better in the long term. The children need to feel able to express their concerns as they are often more aware of the seriousness of the situation than the parents realize. Parents also need to be able to talk with each other and with their children about what is happening and how they feel. The nurse can assess, model, and help to teach communication skills in family work.

Problem-solving skills

Gibson (1988) found that parents of children with cystic fibrosis balanced positive and negative views of the situation and tended to choose the positive view, for example, 'Except for CF, we have a healthy child. There are many children worse than ours'. This positive approach fostered their own coping efforts, enabling them to draw on their own resources and to feel less overwhelmed.

The nurse's role in helping families to cope

Although these strategies have been found to be useful to many families, they are not the answer to everyone's problems. The nurse may need to help families develop the necessary coping strategies that are helpful to *them*. Sensitivity to the needs of the particular family is necessary in order not to create additional stress by suggesting coping strategies they do not consider helpful.

One method of coping can conflict with another. For example, a family may need to be more open in its communication about the illness and the future, but the parents' main preoccupation may be with trying to master the situation and keep control over events. Being forced to talk about their feelings or answer their child's difficult questions may undermine their self-control and ability to cope at that time. Later, when they have come to terms with the illness and do not feel so vulnerable, they may be able to do this. Similarly, parents may not want to discuss the illness in detail with their children as this might conflict with their attempts to pretend the child is well and normal. The nurse can temporarily take over the responsibility from the parents, and talk about the condition with the children.

It is also important to look at family coping strategies from a developmental perspective. As time passes, the family will go through transitions in how they cope with the problem; at different times they will need different amounts of help. The nurse needs to be flexible and patient, and be able to meet the demands of the family when they require it.

A study by Zeitlin and Williamson (1990) attempted to measure the coping behaviours of young disabled children and found they vary markedly in their coping styles and effectiveness. Disabled infants and toddlers' coping is more erratic, less flexible, and more restricted in the range of alternative strategies than non-disabled peers. The least effective area is that of self-initiated coping, which may be due to the different pattern of interaction that develops between a disabled child and their parents. Other research by Wassermand *et al.* (1985) suggests that parents often adopt a more directive interactional pattern in order to stimulate responses from their disabled child, which can produce passivity and inattention.

The role of the specialist nurse in supporting families with chronically sick children is varied and requires a wide range of skills. A study by Moyer (1989) of specialist nurses supporting families with diabetic children compared two groups of parents, one with and one without access to a diabetes nurse specialist (DNS). The topics chosen most frequently for discussion are shown in Table 5.2.

The topic of general medical care was of greatest concern to the parents without a diabetes nurse specialist, while concerns about diet were of more concern to parents with a nurse specialist. The group with a nurse specialist had a broader range of needs that were oriented to the child's normal daily activities growth, and development, rather than being illness focused. Interestingly, the level of parental concerns were about the same in the two groups, and both groups identified their concerns about the children's future as being very important (see Table 5.3).

Table 5.2 *Seven topics chosen most frequently for discussion by parents of diabetic children (Moyer, 1989)*

Topic	% parents needing information	
	Access to diabetic nurse specialist (n = 88)	No access to diabetic nurse specialist (n = 72)
Diet	53	32
Marrying/having children	50	29
Diabetes	36	36
Managing behaviour	36	26
Minor illness	34	38
Emotional development	34	18
Growth/development	33	28
Physical care	21	39

Table 5.3 *Areas of most concern to parents of diabetic children over the previous three months (Moyer, 1989)*

Area of concern	DNS parents (n = 88)	Non-DNS parents (n = 72)
Extra demands on time	26	17
Feeling worn out	24	14
Making child happy	31	27
Taking care of child	25	18
Having money for expenses	25	18
Having adequate agencies in the community	17	16
Wondering about the future	63	47
Responsibility of caring for a child with a worry	31	24

Even though most parents felt that they were coping well with the day-to-day management of diabetes, a large proportion had immediate and ongoing needs for information, help, and support with several aspects of their child's care and development. The nurse specialist did not appear to reduce the level of concern, and it has been suggested that a nurse specialist could foster dependence. However, a nurse specialist may enhance parents' awareness and expectations to achieve near-perfect metabolic control, but this study provides no information on this outcome measure. Alternatively, families may need ongoing support and information on different topics as they gain more skill and competence.

Exercise

When planning support for a family with a six-year-old child with spina bifida, describe three areas of family functioning that the nurse should assess. Explore the use of a care plan in providing care and support for the child at home.

Compliance with treatment

Worry about treatment and medication can significantly affect the parent–child relationship. Normal forgetfulness or carelessness by an ill child may become life-threatening if it involves medication, creating great stress around a common issue of conflict between parents and children. The parents of most healthy adolescents have to negotiate a difficult period of testing of parental control and the transfer of responsibility. When the adolescent is also chronically ill, the issue becomes even more emotionally charged. The mother may feel so anxious that she takes over the responsibility, undermining her child's normal desire for self-control and self-determination (Powers *et al.*, 1984). The adolescent may learn to absolve him or herself of all responsibility for their condition, yet resent or undermine the mother's control. This can lead to a dangerous situation where the adolescent refuses to comply with the treatment, and the condition becomes unstable because of the ongoing fight for control. In this case, the medical condition is compromised through emotional and behavioural conflicts, not through degeneration or medical complications.

Case study

Victoria, aged 16 years, was admitted because of repeated vomiting. An oesophageal repair in babyhood had led to repeated admissions for dilatation of her oesophagus. No organic basis for her vomiting could be found, but nurses observed an over-protective attitude from her mother and socially immature behaviour in Victoria. When her mother left the ward, Victoria would get off her bed and join in ward activities, but when her mother was there she would refuse to get up and would repeatedly retch. The mother demanded residential accommodation in the hospital and it was very difficult for ward staff to keep her off the ward. Eventually the doctors asked the mother to go home, but she refused.

Czajkowski and Koocher (1987) studied the attitudes and coping behaviours of 40 adolescent and young adult patients with cystic fibrosis. They found that measures of attitudes and coping styles could predict compliance to treatment and could significantly discriminate between compliant and non-compliant groups. They used three measures.

1. Participants were asked to complete five stories involving a decision about whether or not to follow medical advice. They were scored along compliance/coping, optimism, and self-efficacy.
2. A questionnaire was used to assess the participant's: medical compliance; severity of illness; future goals; involvement in school or work; openness with peers about the illness; and role in their own medical self-care.
3. A staff questionnaire for the primary medical caregiver (usually the primary nurse) was given to appraise the patient's compliance and optimism during the current hospitalization; and to assess the severity of the illness.

Adolescents who believed their actions made a difference were more likely to deal adaptively with their lives and illness. There was a positive correlation between a health optimism score and medical compliance. Non-compliant adolescents, however, were not overt about their pessimism. They expressed their attitudes in more indirect ways, such as tending to avoid discussion of the future or seeing a no-change situation in their medical condition. Active coping responses reflected a strong emphasis on the value of life; a realistic acceptance of the severity of the illness was a major variable affecting their adaptive functioning.

This type of study provides an important insight into the cognitive and emotional processes operating in chronically ill children and can offer the possibility of predictive intervention to reduce patient morbidity.

Preparing children for hospitalization

Some children still arrive at hospital thinking they are on a special outing to visit granny. Parents are often frightened of telling their child they are going to hospital; they are worried about the child's distress, and fear they may not be able to get the child to leave home. The community nurse is in a position to help parents to understand the best way of preparing their child so the child can cope with the stress. The aim is to help both the child and the parents to adjust psychologically to the impending event and the subsequent emotional changes.

Hospital admission may be very anxiety-provoking for the parents, who at the same time must try to help the child to cope with their own fears. Preparation should therefore take into account the parents' emotional state as well as the child's. A parent who is incapacitated by anxiety will not be able to answer their child's questions, or cope with their worries. They are also likely to communicate their anxiety and make the child even more worried. Parents who try to cover up and say that everything is going to be all right, and yet are clearly upset, can cause the child to think that an unknown and seriously worrying event is about to happen.

The preparation required for each family will be different, and in order to optimize service delivery it is important for the nurse to accurately assess which families require special help. The three main areas of assessment and intervention include:

- the level of anxiety expressed by the parent or child;
- the parents' and child's level of knowledge;
- the type of coping methods used by the parents and child.

Anxiety about going into hospital

Families showing high levels of anxiety, who have little knowledge of what to expect and who cope poorly with stress, will require help. It is still not clear from the research whether including parents in the preparation for their child's hospitalization has any effect on the child's level of stress and ability to cope when they are in hospital; but there is evidence that the parents' emotional state will influence their ability to manage their child.

It is often difficult to assess whether a child is experiencing anxiety as they may not say they are worried, and their behaviour may not reflect their inner state. Assessment of the child's emotional state may need to be done specifically or separately from the parents' and should take into account three main considerations (Zurlinden, 1985).

Age of the child and developmental level

A very young child may not know what going to hospital means and so may not show any anxiety. A junior-age child may be worried about procedures and the strangeness of the situation, and an adolescent may be concerned about personal privacy, the loss of control, and possible pain.

Hazards of hospitalization

Hospital admission can mean different experiences for the child, depending on their illness and the reason for the hospitalization. Some of these experiences can increase the amount of anxiety generated by the admission. These include the level of hurt or injury the child is experiencing or will experience; the strangeness of the environment and hospital staff; separation from home, parents, and siblings; uncertain limits to their behaviour in hospital; loss of control.

Balancing factors

Children who have had bad experiences in hospital are likely to be more frightened than children who have had good experiences. A child who has a lot of social support from the parents, friends, and relatives will not be as frightened as the child who has none at all and feels lonely and isolated. The child's ability to cope with new and different events will also determine the level of anxiety they feel: some see it as an exciting and interesting adventure, while others are worried and frightened.

Parents' and child's level of knowledge

Both children and parents need to know what is going to happen and how it is going to happen. Vague and unclear information is far more upsetting than what is known and understood. Unexpected stress is also more upsetting than expected stress.

Before the admission date the parents may want information about the sequence of events, such as details about the admission procedure; whether they can stay in hospital with the child, and where they will be; what the child can take with them; and special meals prepared to suit their religion, ethnic group, or preference. They may want descriptions of the hospital procedures and routines, or they may want information about what they will see, hear, smell, and feel. Parents may feel more at ease once they know the *practical* details, but children may be more interested in the *sensory* information and how this will affect them.

The admission of a child to hospital is a family crisis. Arrangements have to be made for the whole family: who will care for the other

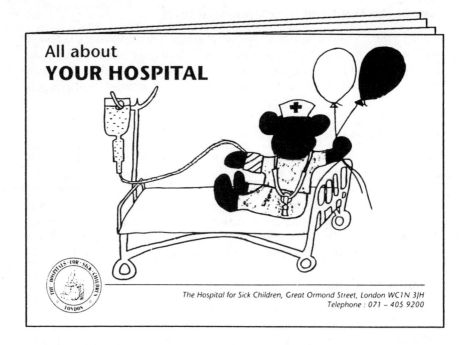

All about
YOUR HOSPITAL

The Hospital for Sick Children, Great Ormond Street, London WC1N 3JH
Telephone : 071 – 405 9200

children if mother goes into hospital with her child? How long will this be for? How will the family get to the hospital for visits? Will mother or father need to take time off work? Is this unpaid time or holiday, and what are the financial implications?

For families from different ethnic backgrounds the prospect may be more worrying because of the cultural change in living arrangements while in hospital. Mothers may be reluctant to talk to male doctors, and may be worried about the need for certain foods or religious observances. Concern about the language barrier may mean that families are reluctant to question what is happening.

Hospitals and clinics across the country have their own preparation materials for going into hospital. There are children's books to read at home, leaflets available from clinics, even pre-admission visits to the hospital may be possible. Action for Sick Children also provide leaflets and information for parents and children. There is often general information that can be given to parents to read at home, but there are always individual concerns as well, and parents may need a chance to talk about these.

The reason for giving information is usually to help the parents and child to cope better with the impending change. The giving of information itself is usually helpful. In some children, the knowledge may actually heighten anxiety – termed 'anticipatory anxiety' – but

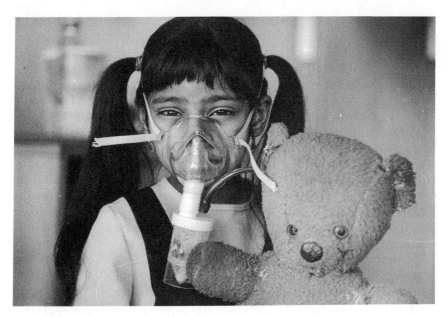

© Camilla Jessel and Action for Sick Children. Reproduced by permission.

this too can be beneficial in helping the child to cope better when the stress actually occurs. However, the child's age and level and quality of previous experience of hospitals and medical staff are important in how effective any preparation will be.

Because children under the age of seven often have difficulty understanding time, preparation that occurs too early may be of no help at all. While the older child will be able to understand that a hospital admission is a month or more away, a young child only needs to be told the day before, or on the day. Children benefit from being told the reason for them having to go to hospital, but this should be linked to the child's level of understanding and language. Reasons should be stated in positive and reassuring ways. The child may want to know practical details, such as which toy they can take with them, or whether they can wear their own pyjamas, and where they are going to sleep.

Types of coping methods

Some families have a self-protective mechanism of denying or trying to forget that the child is going to hospital, and so do not talk about the event or prepare for it. In this way, anxiety is kept at a low level. They wait until the last possible minute to anticipate what is going to happen, and even then may not tell the child until he or she is at the door of the hospital for fear of upsetting them. In some circumstances this may be an adaptive way of coping, particularly if the admission date is a long time away, the child is very young, or the admission date could be changed. However, in families where there is a lot of anxiety about the admission, this is not the best way of coping as there is no opportunity for the fears to be expressed and worked out, information cannot be requested, and lack of knowledge is therefore perpetuated.

Other families make great efforts to prepare for the hospitalization, including the heightening of the level of anxiety about the admission. Parents and children may talk about it openly, read books to the child about going into hospital, and may visit the hospital. They may tell all of their friends and relatives, and openly make preparations for the family while the child is away. Such a family may show good adaptation to the anticipated event, but then feel let down if the admission date is delayed or postponed.

Some families develop good mechanisms in order to cope with the anxiety. They may use social support, seek knowledge, or develop an effective and open communication system between family members so that they can share their feelings and reassure each other. If the anxiety is denied or ridiculed, then that member of the family may have no way of coping with their worries, and may have to turn to external support, or try to develop their own individual coping methods.

Helping families to cope with hospital admission

Some children may need intensive and active help to learn how to cope effectively with their fears and worries. Children and parents who feel very anxious prior to a hospital admission might benefit from learning some behavioural techniques to reduce anxiety. Not all families will need this, but there are some at-risk children and parents. One mother may be more of a worrier or generally more anxious than another, her previous experiences of ineffectively managing stress having accumulated to influence her present level of anxiety. She may require support to express her concerns, and then how to manage them. Teaching her some relaxation exercises to practise in association with thinking about the hospital and the imminent admission may help her, in turn, to be a more effective supporter of her child (Zastowny *et al.*, 1986).

The parent and child can benefit from practising coping skills together, for example when the parent is given the role of a 'coping teacher', who teaches the child how to cope. This involves learning how to prepare for stress, how to confront and handle the immediate stress, how to cope with feelings at critical moments, and how to congratulate oneself for coping. Techniques of relaxation, distraction, pleasant thoughts, and images can all be used (Manion, 1990).

Personal discussion time for children or anxiety management training is expensive in regard to professional time, and working with children in groups may be a more cost-effective method. This may be carried out in the hospital as a general introduction for children, or as a specific programme geared to a particular procedure or illness. The family coping methods for dealing with anxiety and stress are also important. Working with the parents to develop coping strategies in the family can be a very effective way of helping them to help their child. If the illness is likely to require repeated admissions, then preparation of the whole family will be essential for an adaptive and flexible approach.

Summary

The psychological care of the sick child in the community involves not only the needs of the child but also of the whole family. It is therefore important to view the management of the child's illnesses as part of a family process: members of the family are affected by the child's condition and, in turn, the way in which the family copes will affect the course of some illnesses. Preparing children and families for hospitalization of the child may also be part of the community nurse's role, particularly where the chronic illness results in repeated admissions that may culminate in increasing fear and distress.

Further reading

Eiser, C. (1990). *Chronic Childhood Disease. An Introduction to Psychological Theory and Research*. Cambridge, Cambridge University Press.
A very readable and comprehensive book that covers most of the issues faced by families and nurses caring for children with chronic disease.

Knafl, K. A. and Deatrick, J. A. (1990). Family management style: concept analysis and development. *Journal of Pediatric Nursing*, 5, 4–14.
Presents a useful and practical outline of how to assess the coping of families with chronically ill children. The issue of the journal has several related articles, all of which are well worth reading.

6 Care of sick children in hospital

The effects of hospital admission

Going into hospital can be one of the most traumatic experiences of a child's life. It may be the first time the child realizes his or her parents cannot stop unpleasant things happening to them; it may be their first experience of real pain and discomfort, or the first time the child has stayed away from home. The child may feel unwell, and therefore less able to cope with the changes and demands of a new place and new people.

The effects of admission are not necessarily negative, particularly as hospitals have become more child-centred, and staff more aware of children's special emotional needs. A single admission for a short time has not been found to have any detrimental effects on children's behavioural and emotional development. While many children show some behavioural reaction to short admissions, particularly if their parents are not admitted with them, these usually disappear in a few weeks (Rutter, 1981); even if the difficult behaviour lasts longer, the child's behaviour is usually back to normal after about six months (Fletcher, 1981). Repeated admissions, however, increase the risk of longer-term effects, especially if the first admission is before the child is five, and if the child comes from a disadvantaged background (Quinton and Rutter, 1976).

The number of times a young child is admitted to hospital after age two and before the age of five is associated with higher levels of anxiety and anti-social behaviour at age five (Haslum, 1988). There is also a strong association between the number of admissions between the ages of five and ten and behaviour at age ten. Admission is a factor that can affect the child's future, as children can be made more vulnerable or more resilient by the experience.

Sylva and Stein (1990) have identified the following features that affect children's reactions to hospitalization:

- the child's temperamental characteristics;
- the frequency and length of hospitalizations;
- the severity and chronicity of the illness;
- the support of the family;
- the type of preparation the child receives.

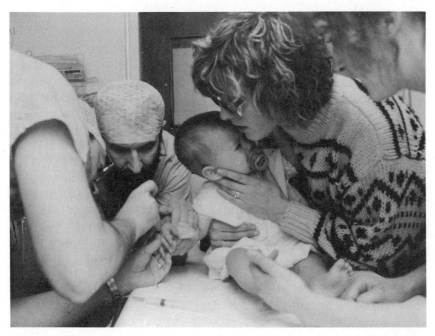

© Royal Manchester Children's Hospital, Camilla Jessel and Action for Sick Children. Reproduced by permission.

The number of stressful procedures the child experiences while in hospital may be the most significant factor in determining the level of distress (Saylor *et al.*, 1987). In terms of affecting medical and nursing attitudes, this knowledge could reduce the number of invasive investigations or painful procedures the child has to experience. The number of potentially painful or stressful procedures indicates how quickly a cumulative stress effect can build up. It is important to limit these experiences as much as possible. The recent trend towards shorter admissions and day cases may help to offset some of the negative effects of hospitalization. The nurse may be the only person who notices the effect of the number or the stressfulness of the procedures on the child, and may be able to suggest alternative ways of attaining the same goal.

Activity

Either observe or ask a colleague who is nursing on an oncology ward to list the number of potential stressors on the first admission of a five-year-old with leukaemia. Take care to consider every aspect of the child's care. Consider emotional stressors, i.e. separation from family, pets, home; environmental stress, i.e. access to play area and toys, movement of bed, noise, ward events; as well as the stress of medical and nursing procedures.

Helping children with admission to hospital

A child's initial impressions when he or she first comes into hospital are important. Ideally a designated nurse, or the nurse who met the parents in outpatients, will welcome the family to the ward. The nurse should know who the parents are, the child's name, and why the child has been admitted. A bed should be ready for the child to go to so that a 'personal' area is immediately allocated to the family. Helping the child and the parents to understand the layout of the ward and the systems easily and without undue stress is one way of enabling them to feel co-operative and calm. The nurse's smile, welcome, and the time taken to explain procedures and to orient the family are invaluable. The parents need to feel welcomed and settled so that they can reassure their child and help him or her to cope with the new surroundings. Both the parents and the child may have many unanswered questions about practical issues, for example whether the child can wear their own night clothes, or how to cope with dietary preferences or restrictions. Each family wants to have its individuality recognized; they often fear they will be sucked into an impersonal system with a pace and process of its own.

Case study

James, aged two years, always had his muslin nappy to cuddle at night and was very particular about having one particular teat on his bottle. His mother was worried that nurses may not realize his preferences and might upset him after his operation by offering a ward bottle instead of his own.

A child who has been experiencing emotional tension at home may be less able to cope with the additional stress of coming into hospital. Important life events like moving house or school, a new baby, parents separating, loss or bereavement, will all upset children's normal ability to adapt and cope.

Exercise
What everyday concerns might an Asian family have about their six-year-old son coming into hospital? What ten questions should the nurse ask the parents to find out about their child's special needs and preferences? (Suggested answers at end of book.)

Parents on the ward

The hospital should recognize the child as a member of a family, whose support during the hospital stay is essential to the child's well being. The hospital should also enable parents to give love, care, comfort, and support to their child, especially at the most stressful times, for example during and after treatment, induction of anaesthesia, investigation and X-rays.

Unrestricted visiting

There has been an immense revolution in medical and nursing attitudes over the last 20 years in relation to unrestricted visiting. Nurses have been able to realize and incorporate a totally new view of the role of parents during the admission of their child to hospital. The Department of Health Report (1991) specifies that there should be unrestricted parental involvement during the child's hospital stay, and that parents and members of the immediate family should be encouraged and assisted to be with the child at all times, unless the medical interests of the child preclude this.

Parents of young children are expected to stay in hospital with their children during the admission, if there is accommodation available, or have unrestricted visiting of their child. A number of studies demonstrate that children benefit from having their parents near them during this time of uncertainty and stress. One study showed that children admitted with their parents for tonsillectomy were less likely to have postoperative complications or infections than children in a control group who were admitted without their parents (Brain and Maclay, 1968). The importance of their presence for the child should be made clear to the parents so they can decide whether to stay in or not.

Parental care on the ward

In the United States, 'Care-by-Parent' schemes have extended the role of parents on the ward so that the resident parent agrees to be responsible for the care of their child while in hospital. The nurses teach the parents routine nursing procedures, which are then recorded and carried out by the parents. The nurses are available for consultation, but are not routinely present. The types of patients considered suitable for this type of care include:

• Children whose nursing care is minimal, or of the kind that any parent would normally be expected to carry out.

- Children whose condition is long-term, and specific techniques of observation or treatment must be learned and carried out at home if the child is to live at home.
- Families that require general health education, including diet, hygiene, or child-rearing practices to lessen the likelihood of deterioration in the child's condition or recurring episodes of illness.

The most important criterion in this scheme was the willingness of the parents to participate fully (Lerner *et al.*, 1972).

The scheme has been replicated in Britain by Cleary *et al.* (1986), who carried out an observational study and demonstrated differences between parents in the care-by-parent scheme; resident parents not in the scheme; and non-resident parents. The greatest difference was in the length of hospital stay: children without resident parents had longer-than-average stays. Other results indicated significant differences in sleeping and crying, and how often the child was alone when awake. Children without resident parents slept more than the other two groups. More striking, children without a resident parent were awake alone three times as often as the group with a resident parent, and the children of resident parents were awake alone nearly three times as often as children in the care-by-parent scheme. The study demonstrated that children without a resident parent lack the warm, social atmosphere a family can provide, while children in the care-by-parent scheme have more opportunity for social interaction, and have 90% of their interactions with family members, particularly mothers. And, on examining the nursing care of the parents, nurses rated the parents as being very capable of providing a good level of care (Sainsbury *et al.*, 1986).

The nurse is no longer just caring for the sick child, but may also have to care for the parents. The nurse needs to negotiate with and tell parents what is expected of them during their child's stay on the ward. They may need to be taught and helped to learn how to carry out simple monitoring procedures, or how to help look after their child. They may need to be made aware of their responsibilities, and that they are there for the sake of the child. This type of scheme is not prevalent in Britain today, but it may mark the way for a more active role for parents during their child's admission in the future.

Parents' privacy

It is very unwelcoming to parents to only have an uncomfortable chair by the child's bed to sit on; to have to go to the hospital canteen every time to get a drink or something to eat; and to feel continually under public observation, with no privacy to express their grief, anxiety, or stress. Parents are often forced to walk the streets outside the hospital to cry if they do not want their child to see how upset they feel. Parents

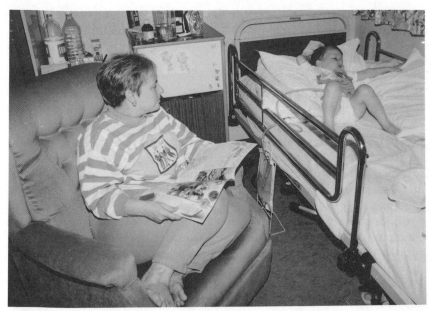

© Alder Hey Hospital, Liverpool, Elisabeth Hommel and Action for Sick Children. Reproduced by permission.

need their own area which they can retire to if stressed or over-tired, where they can drink, eat, or use the telephone. If they are to be accepted as part of every young child's admission, then thought and preparation needs to be given to helping the parents to feel settled so that they can support their child. It is not enough to change hospital policy to unrestricted visiting or providing beds for parents and yet continue to provide the same facilities available 20 years ago to parents who would visit only two hours a day.

Supporting the parents

Paediatric nurses must be good communicators and listeners in order to support the parents. Many parents express their worries and concerns to nurses. It takes time and effort to cope with the desperation and anguish some parents feel; it can be very draining on the nurse's energy and emotions. Some parents may be so anxious that they make continual demands on nursing time to talk over the same problems repeatedly; others cope by becoming aggressive and awkward. Nurses need to provide adequate time for each family, regardless of their demands, particularly if there are cultural differences or a reluctance to complain or to say anything.

Nurses may be asked to interpret comments or diagnoses made by medical staff into language the parents can understand. Some nurses go round to the parents after the doctor's ward round to explain what has been said and to help parents deal with their feelings.

Separation from the parents

If parents are unable to stay in hospital with their child, either for family reasons or through a lack of accommodation in the hospital, it is important for them not to feel in any way condemned. Although parental presence is generally good for the child's welfare, it is possible for nurses to make parents feel guilty when it is not possible for them to stay if, for example, the children at home may have nobody to look after them, or the pressures of work or other responsibilities may be too great.

Children who have experienced happy and brief separations from their parents before the hospital admission are likely to be more able to cope with their parents not staying than a child who has never had that experience; they will have experienced 'stress immunization' (Stacey *et al.*, 1970). The age of the child also has an effect: the younger the child, the more need there is for the parent to stay, although when Ross and Ross (1984) asked five to twelve-year-olds what would have helped them most when they were experiencing the worst pain, almost without exception the children said having their parents with them.

The nurse has to tread a fine line between welcoming and encouraging parents to stay, and understanding when they cannot. Helping the parents to work out visiting schedules whereby other members of the family or friends and relatives visit the child when they cannot is one way of enabling the parents to realize the importance of family contact, but also recognizes the other demands in their lives. Parents can also alternate visiting, and share the responsibility and time involved. Children who are able to maintain contacts with life outside at home and at school seem better able to cope with the effects of being in hospital.

Anxious parents

The way in which parents relate to their child has marked effect on the child's understanding of what is happening, and also on their ability to cope. Some parents may be reluctant to tell their child what is happening because they are worried about frightening them, so losing the opportunity to help their child prepare for the stresses and pain that might occur. Or they may be so protective that they do not allow the child to develop an appropriate level of autonomy in coping with what is happening. Parents who are frightened and worried may communicate their anxiety to their child, and exacerbate any fears that already exist. Poor communication between the parents and child may also have this effect, as without the correct information, the child's worries may grow.

Despite these occasional difficulties, most evidence points to the immensely positive effect that parental presence has on the young child's ability to cope in hospital.

Adolescents on the ward

Adolescents are usually misplaced either in a ward with adult patients, or on a young children's ward. Preferably, they should be in a ward with other young adults of the same age. If this is not possible, the adolescent can be placed in a cubicle in order to give him or her some privacy and personal space.

Adolescence is a difficult age to be a patient as the role conflicts with the pressures to grow up and be independent; being a patient forces them into being dependent and controlled by others in authority. They may feel like regressing because they are unwell, yet find this hard to do because their relationship with their parents has altered. They may feel they can't have the cuddle they really want, or the parents may not realize that this is what is needed.

Adolescents are also coping with changing bodies and feelings. As sexual development progresses they may feel unusually sensitive to physical investigations or procedures. They may be shy and find undressing for examinations difficult. They deserve the respect and considerations of modesty shown an adult, rather than considering them as unselfconscious children.

Personal care

While adolescents can be taught to do many procedures for themselves, they may fluctuate in their compliance or desire to carry them out. This may indicate an assertion of identity, self-control or an abdication of any responsibility. Helping the adolescent to feel a sense of control over themselves and what happens to them is important in order to gain their co-operation and to maintain their precarious sense of identity. Self-monitoring methods using charts or checklists, and involving them in formulating their own plan of care, can enable the adolescent to gain a sense of control. This needs to be done through negotiation and understanding, not through bullying and irritation. It is easy to take an authoritarian role, but this often will not work because the problems are based in the adolescents' reaction to precisely that issue. Finding out what they think about the situation and their point of view is essential in gaining their co-operation.

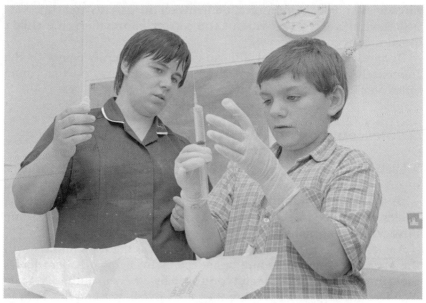

© Elisabeth Hommel and Action for Sick Children. Reproduced by permission.

Positive feedback and attention

Adolescence is a time of intense feelings and conflicts. The individual is trying to understand their feelings, and also to develop their own values and attitudes. It is a time of testing out different types of reactions and behaviour. Giving the adolescent feedback about the effects of their behaviour can be one way of increasing their awareness of others' reactions as they need to understand the limits to their behaviour, and to respect the needs of other patients and parents on the ward.

Building trust

The adolescent may feel anxious and concerned about their condition. Taking time to talk and understand their feelings is important in helping the teenage child to cope with being in hospital. They might understand rationally what is happening to them, but have not had the chance to deal with their emotional reactions to the situation.

Case study

Simon (aged 15 years) required an amputation of his leg after a road traffic accident. Initially he was just happy to be alive and his parents could only focus on that issue. But after the amputation, as he started to recover, he became withdrawn and depressed. He felt unable to talk to his parents – he had disobeyed them by riding his bike on the main road. The friends who had visited him had been noisy and cracked jokes. He needed the nurses to take time to talk over what happened, and the possibilities for his future and his sense of shame and guilt at the accident.

Some can discuss their feelings with their parents, while others can't, so it is important for the nurse to determine how much support the adolescent is receiving from friends and relatives. Adolescents can be very good at covering up their feelings and pretending that everything is all right. They need to develop a trusting relationship with the nurse, which requires time, genuine interest, and a concern for their feelings and experiences. They also require an openness from the nurse and the freedom to discuss their concerns about their treatment and condition.

Setting limits

It may be appropriate to give the adolescent more independence than is usual on a children's ward. Some may want to help out and look after the younger children, while others may just want to be left alone on their beds. Some may be concerned about examinations at school, and want the time and space to study. Setting well-defined limits about behaviour on the ward helps the adolescent to understand what is permissible, and to develop a sense of security and confidence in the staff.

Group involvement

Adolescents often want to be part of a group, and the process of hospitalization singles them out as being different. Helping them talk about their concerns, and suggesting how they might talk to others about their hospitalization can help. For example, they may be worried about how the treatment will affect them when they leave hospital, or later in life. Encouraging them to have their friends visit, or to use the telephone to maintain contact, can help overcome some of the fear and isolation they may feel. They may show signs of depression and apathy, and may miss their friends immensely.

If the adolescent's illness has any implications for their ability to lead a full and normal life, these issues must be broached while they are in hospital. In particular, it is essential to discuss implications for sexual activity or reproductive capacity openly and fully. Adolescents have every right to know about themselves and their body's functioning. During such discussions, it is important to emphasize their strengths

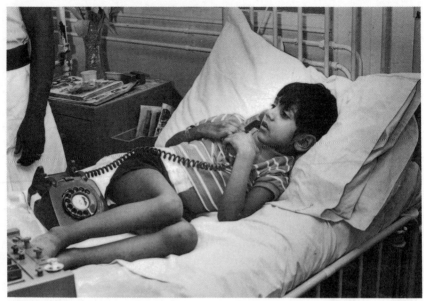

© Camilla Jessel and Action for Sick Children. Reproduced by permission.

and abilities rather than their disabilities, and to teach them how to care for themselves as much as possible.

The long-stay child

Some children stay in hospital for up to a year or more. During this time they are often well and active, but need to be continually monitored medically. Such long-stay patients present a particular problem to the acute style of service offered in most hospitals. The problems facing long-stay children are the same as those for children brought up in group-care residential settings: institutionalization and socially precocious behaviour.

Some young toddlers may never have been home during their first years of life, or they may have only been home for short periods. Although parents may visit regularly, they may be unable to stay in hospital for the length of the child's admission. The child becomes a semi-permanent fixture on the ward, making very close and dependent relationships with the staff. This is sometimes so intense that nurses can feel in competition with the parents for the affection of the child. While it is important for the child's psychological health to be able to make such attachments, unfortunately nursing allocation and staffing means that many nurses are transient on the wards, and so the child has to get to know new staff repeatedly. The ward sister and the occasional long-stay staff nurse are the most permanent staff members on a ward, and are extremely important people for the child.

Non-resident parents should be encouraged to maintain their relationship with the child, and be aware of the child's developmental progress. Parents need to understand any behavioural changes that are occurring, and nurses should discuss with them the management of the child on the ward. Here, clear communication is important: as the ward sister acts in place of the parents, ultimate decisions about management of the child's behaviour are made by her.

Keeping the parents and child in touch over these very long periods can be a strain. The family is stressed by continual visiting, the costs of travelling, and having a dislocated family. With older children, regular telephoning is a great help. If parents are not able to visit often, then it may be necessary to suggest that a social 'aunt' visits – in some hospitals a local person from the nearby community will come regularly to visit the child. Keeping a special relationship going over a long period is important in the development of the child's sense of identity in the rapidly changing ward environment.

Play and education

Play is essential to the intellectual, social, and emotional development of children. It can help them resolve stressful situations, reduce anxiety, facilitate communication, and speeds recovery and rehabilitation.

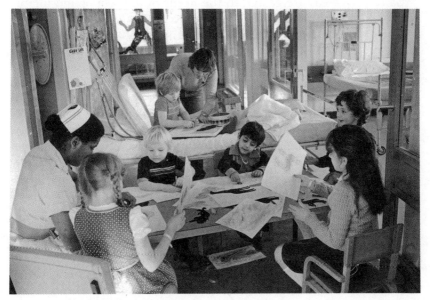

© Action for Sick Children. Reproduced by permission.

Hospitals should employ play specialists or nursery nurses specifically to play with the children and keep them happy and well-occupied. They will plan the play area and arrange for special creative and messy activities to take place such as modelling, painting, or sticking. The organization of play materials and experiences is important in order to ensure that the children are fully occupied during the day, and that their interest is maintained.

Bolig (1984) has identified five main functions of play in hospital: to provide diversion; to play out problems and anxieties; to restore normal aspects of life; to aid understanding of hospital events; and to communicate fear. One study examined the type of play pre-school children used to reduce anxiety on their first day at school. It demonstrated that highly anxious children appear to benefit from the opportunity to play, and tend to engage in more dramatic and fantasy play in contrast to low-anxiety children, who show more functional and constructional play. The study also demonstrated that highly anxious children are better able to resolve their anxiety through playing alone rather than with peers.

During their play, children need to have their concentration extended. They also require a trusted and responsive adult present to help occupy them. The play specialist should not take part in any painful or medical procedures, and so becomes a safety haven for children who are enduring unpleasant procedures. They may form a special relationship with a child, providing extra emotional support during the child's admission.

Many play areas are geared to the needs of pre-school and infant-aged children, but school-age children also need educational activities, arranged by the hospital teacher. It is important to minimize the disruptive effect of hospitalization on normal life, and so they need to keep up with their age group in school work. Hospital-based teachers will provide work suitable to the child's age range, or will contact the child's school to find out what they should be doing. If a child is not feeling well, then they clearly cannot concentrate or perform well, but they should be given the opportunity to work if they want to. For secondary-age children, the worry of examinations can cause additional stress, and allowing them the chance to study will relieve this anxiety. Parents can contact the child's school to bring in the necessary books and work; visiting friends will also bring in information about school and what the patient should be doing.

Adolescents may be unsure of their feelings, but help with their school work can be the start of a trusting relationship. They enjoy adult attention and interest in what they are doing. They may need help to complete a task, or they will want to show what they have done. Taking time to watch, provide advice or help, and to praise achievements are all essential parts of good nursing care.

The needs of the whole child must be recognized. Taking time in the nursing plan to provide the psychological and emotional care that children require is essential, and can make a children's ward a happy and relaxing place for the children and staff.

Exercise

Make a list of play materials that might help pre-school children to work through their anxieties while in hospital. (Suggested answers at end of book.)

The child's understanding of illness

In order for children to understand information about their illness or treatment, it is necessary first to identify their level of understanding of how the body works. Eiser and Patterson (1983) carried out a simple study investigating children's ideas about the inside of their bodies. They asked six-, eight-, ten-, and twelve-year-old children to: draw the inside of their bodies; draw a circle around the heart, brain, stomach, lungs, kidney, liver, and bladder on an outline diagram provided; and describe the function of these organs; explain which parts of their body were needed to eat, breathe, get rid of waste, and swim.

They found an increase in the number of body parts mentioned at increasing ages, but the mean number mentioned by each age group was lower than other reported studies in the United States. The most frequently mentioned were the brain (76%), heart (74%), bones (71%), blood (58%), and lungs (38%). Only two children mentioned sexual or reproductive organs. The children's explanation of the function of body parts increased in sophistication with age, but few children knew the purpose of the bladder or the liver. Their ideas about the interconnection of body parts in bodily functions, for example the link between eating and the circulatory system, was not made even by twelve-year-olds while six-year-olds had little awareness of where food went after it left their stomachs.

When a seven-year-old girl was asked what specific parts of her body were for she answered:

'If you didn't have your heart you'd die because it keeps you alive. I don't know how it keeps you alive. If you aren't very well the doctors can tell with a special thing. When they put the thing in their ears they can hear the heart thumping.
If you didn't have your brain you can't think what you want to be

when you grow up. Your brain helps you because it sends messages to your ears to listen – there could be a car coming.

If you didn't have your stomach you couldn't go to the loo and you'd never eat anything because you wouldn't feel hungry.

Your lungs look like two big balloons; they help you to breathe; you couldn't stay alive without them.

(Kidneys) From your stomach they go down to there and you can go to the toilet when it's full up.

(Bladder) Is that something near your bottom? What is it?'

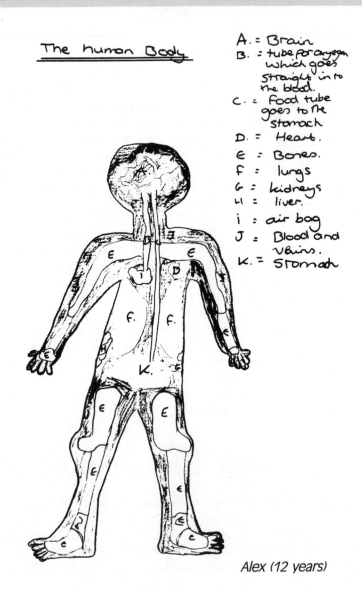

The human Body

A. = Brain
B. = tube for oxygen which goes straight into the blood.
C. = Food tube goes to the stomach
D. = Heart.
E. = Bones.
f = lungs
G = kidneys
H = liver.
i = air bag
J = Blood and veins.
k. = Stomach

Alex (12 years)

MY Body

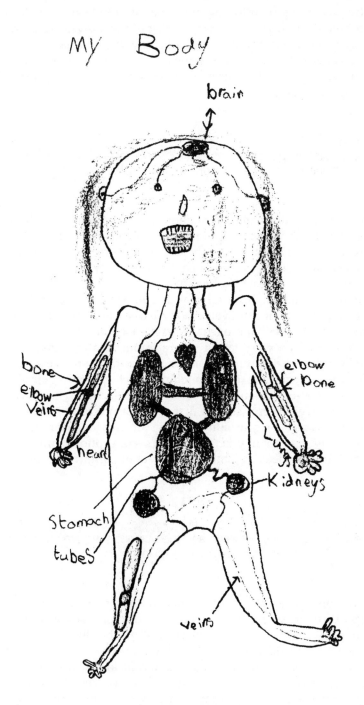

Amanda (7 years)

The frequency of mentioning the role of the heart and lungs in breathing increased with age, while most of the six-year-olds and half of the eight-year-olds could not describe how the body got rid of waste. Younger children thought the bones caused their limbs to move in swimming, while older children acknowledged the role of the brain in controlling movement.

Activity
It would be interesting to repeat the study by Eiser and Patterson (1983) on children of different ages for your own information and understanding.

It is helpful if children are taught about their anatomy and physiology before they are faced with an impending event such as hospitalization or surgery, but it may be left to the doctor or nurse to explain how the body works to recently admitted children. A study that examined two different methods of teaching healthy young children aged four-and-a-half to seven-and-a-half found that a multisensory approach using a life-size rag doll with removable body parts was more effective than the more traditional approach of using two-dimensional pictures. When the children were tested several months later, those who had learned via the rag doll remembered significantly more (Vessey, 1988).

How the nurse progresses on to telling the child about their illness or impending surgery should be based on the child's cognitive and intellectual level. Nurses should first find out precisely how the child views the cause of the illness and the reasons for treatment. Explanations can then take the child's conceptions into account, introducing new ideas to match their level of comprehension.

Exercise
Think how you would explain to a five-year-old, who has never been in hospital before, about his hernia and the operation required to repair it. What would you use to illustrate your explanation?

Some research studies have found that children's conceptions of illness progress through stages that match their thinking about other topics (Perrin and Gerrity, 1981; Brewster, 1982). The difficulty here is in defining levels of cognitive development in terms of chronological age: children of the same age will show different levels of understanding depending on their experiences and differing ranges of information.

Young children often associate illness with justice: children under the age of seven often consider the onset of illness as the outcome of wrongdoing. Young children are likely to extend the concept of contagion to include non-contagious illness and accidents, and accept immanent justice as an explanation for illness and accident. But as they grow older and develop a more advanced understanding of contagion, their use of the concept of immanent justice decreases (Kister and Patterson, 1980).

In examining how 50 chronically ill hospitalized children between the ages of five and thirteen understood the cause of their illness, the reasons for treatment, and the role of medical personnel in providing treatment, Brewster (1982) found a three-stage sequence of conceptual development:

1. Illness is caused by human action (the under 7 age group).
2. Illness is due to physical causality, e.g., germs (usually the 7 to 10 age group).
3. Illness has multiple causes and is caused by interactions of events (over 9 age group).

Case study

When Kelly (aged six) was asked why she had headaches, she replied, 'Because I think too hard'. Her sister, aged 11 years said, 'It's because Mummy and Daddy fight and the baby cries so much'.

A parallel three-stage sequence of understanding the intent of medical procedures included:

1. The child views the procedures as punishment.
2. The child correctly perceives the intent of the procedures, but believes staff empathy depends on the expression of pain.
3. The child can infer both intention and empathy from staff.

The questions that remain unanswered are whether better explanations of illness could result in better understanding by the child, and whether such understanding could result in better adjustment to, and coping with, the illness.

Activity
We rarely ask children about what they think caused their illness as we are usually too involved with telling them. During your time on a children's ward take some time to ask each child about what caused their illness and note the replies, together with the age of the child. This will provide some fascinating first-hand information about children's thought processes and concepts at different ages.

The child's ability to cope with stress

Each child is an individual and will have different ways of coping with stress. The accurate prediction of coping is dependent on such individual differences, but is also related to different stressors, different coping processes, and the outcome of coping. Attempts to measure children's coping is complicated by their rapidly changing perceptions and abilities as they develop.

Children's ability to recognize a stressor is dependent on their developmental level. To understand the significance of the stressor, the child needs to be able to remember previous similar experiences, and to predict when the event will happen. Memories of past stressful medical events may be absent or distorted, and their poor understanding of time will limit their ability to evaluate the importance of the ensuing event; they are also subject to cognitive distortions and erroneous beliefs, for example, that diabetes is caused by eating too much sugar or that their blood will leak out through a vein puncture. Coping processes have a number of different facets: •

- Active, or information-seeking, versus passive, or avoidant, coping methods: i.e. children who ask questions, want to touch equipment and watch procedures versus those who hide their faces, won't look at staff and refuse to touch equipment.
- Internal versus external coping methods: i.e., children who use guided imagery, hypnosis and relaxation versus those who cry out loud, want distraction and play with preparatory materials.
- Emotionally-focused versus problem-focused coping methods: i.e. children who learn to control and express their feelings versus those who cope by using problem-solving.

The relationship between these facets has not been fully investigated yet.

Peterson (1989) has reviewed a number of studies examining active versus avoidant coping in children. In general, children who are active copers seem to manage the stress better than avoiders. Less defensive children tend to play with medically relevant toys; and those children who select medically relevant toys prior to hospitalization also have lower levels of self-reported anxiety following hospitalization. Active copers are less anxious, more co-operative, and have a higher tolerance for pain than children who are passive copers.

The diversity in methods of conceptualizing and measuring children's coping indicates a need for greater consensus in this research area. Actively seeking information, like watching a procedure or asking questions, is not necessarily the same as deliberately using a psychologically active (but physically passive) strategy, such as imagery, self-instruction, or relaxation. Measures of coping are also unclear at present: some advocate self-report measures while others measure observable behaviours. A boy who deliberately relaxes is using a different coping strategy from a boy who is physically limp in hopelessness and resignation, although they look physically similar.

Actively coping children respond well to explanations about what is happening; to 'show and tell' techniques; and to opportunities to indicate when the pain is getting to be too much. They benefit from play preparation, discussion, and information, using the opportunities to work out what is going to happen on dolls and teddies, and actively joining in hospital play. Such children will touch hospital equipment and familiarize themselves with gowns, masks, and syringes; they read preparation material, watch films, and ask questions. What is not clear is whether active copers recover faster because of their personalities, or whether the preparatory information helps them (LaMontagne, 1987).

Until recently, the general assumption was that all children benefit from developmentally appropriate preparation, but this is now being questioned. Children who are avoiders may find preparation detrimental to their coping style: preparation may heighten their anxiety to such a level that they become less able to cope than if not given the information. It is not yet clear how best to help children who are avoiders. Unfortunately, they seem to suffer more after the event, and there is some evidence that even if they are prepared for the procedure their recovery is not enhanced in any way. Whether this is part of the child's personality and is a way in which they keep their arousal at a manageable level, or whether it is a style of coping they have learned from the family, is not yet clear.

Preparation for medical procedures

There are a number of factors that any preparation of children for medical procedures should take into account.

Previous hospital experiences

Understanding the child's past experiences is vital in tailoring preparation to the child's needs. There is some evidence to suggest that giving information to a young child who has previously experienced surgery is likely to heighten their anxiety levels and over-sensitize them (Melamed *et al.*, 1983). Listening to what children enjoyed about a previous admission helps the nurse to understand the experience from the child's point of view, and some of the ideas could be incorporated into the management of the child while on the ward.

Level of anxiety

A child who is very anxious needs to have their level of anxiety reduced before receiving additional anxiety-provoking information in preparation for an operation. Helping them to feel settled on the ward, giving them some control, and establishing a trusting relationship with them will all help.

Preparatory information

This needs to be geared to the age, developmental level, and knowledge of the child. The language used should reflect the child's ability, and the information should reflect the child's concerns. A young child may be concerned about smell and sounds, while an older child may want details about the operation. The young child may want to know where their parents will be and where they will wake up, while an older child may want to know how large the incision will be, and whether they might wake up during the operation. Nurses should be conscious of finding out what the child wants to know rather than concentrating on telling the child what they think the child wants to know.

Case study

Stephen, aged three-and-a-half, was due to have a colostomy. His mother had told him that he would have a small hole made in his tummy for his poo to come out. It would mean he would not have to wear nappies any more and stop his sore bottom. He kept saying 'not now' to the nurses on the ward and although the operation was planned for four days' time, they were able to reassure him that it was 'not now'. The play leader gave him a teddy with a colostomy to play with and, when the day came, he was ready to have his operation 'like teddy'. When his mother told him that she would be there while he had his 'magic sleep' and would be holding his hand when he woke up again, he was much happier.

Involvement of the parents

Parents can take an active role in preparing the child, or they may want to leave this to the nurses. It is important that the parents understand what is going to happen, but sometimes because their knowledge is limited, they may not know how to express this so that their child will understand. In other families, the parents are the best people to talk to their child. It is often helpful, however, if a nurse listens in on the conversation, so that he or she can help with any awkward questions. Playleaders often have special toys and equipment for children and parents to play with and explore what they have been told. Many parents have misconceptions about the outcome of an operation and it is often helpful for them to talk to another child (and parents) with experience of a similar operation.

Case study

Daniel, aged 6, was well prepared for his ileostomy and his mother was looking forward to clean pants and clean beds. But after the operation his mother was shocked and distressed by the look of the ileostomy site and regretted having agreed to the operation. This made Daniel anxious and worried, so he refused to look at the ileostomy or to touch it. It took them both four days to come to terms with the ileostomy and begin to accept it.

The coping style of the child

Nurses can offer to tell children what is going to happen and provide play materials for young children to use if they want to. However, this should not be encouraged if a child is showing resistance or increased stress by listening to, or looking at, what is being offered. Nurses should be sensitive to the reactions of the child, keep stress low but leave preparatory materials around so that the child can approach them in their own time and at their own speed.

Timing of the preparation

Young children are best prepared very close to the event, while older children can be told in advance. Many hospitals have preparatory packages for parents and children, which may be written or on video. These might save nursing time, and if used at home may increase the parents' understanding of their child's concerns and needs. They could, however, create unnecessary fear and anxiety, or they may simply not be used and so may not be cost-effective.

Wolfer and Visintainer (1979) evaluated the stress-reducing effect of the following different types of preparatory methods on five experimental groups of children for tonsillectomy:

☐ Home preparatory materials, including a written and illustrated children's booklet; a hospital kit including a surgical mask, syringe (without a needle), sticking plaster, a rubber band to simulate a

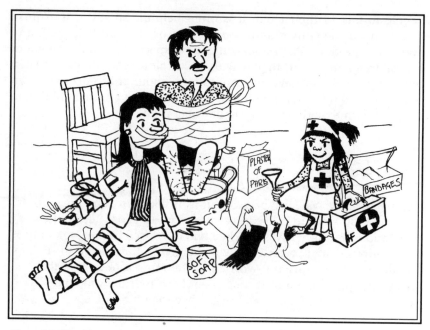

'I'm beginning to doubt the value of parental involvement in preparatory hospital experience.'

tourniquet, an alcohol sponge, a cardboard mask and paper bag to simulate an anaesthetic mask and bag; and an instruction booklet for parents. These were given one week before admission.

☐ Stress-point preparation in hospital by a nurse. Children and parents were given systematic information about the purpose, meaning, and timing of events; information about the sensory experiences the child would have during and following procedures; rehearsal exercises for children to become familiar with procedures, equipment, and their own roles and responses during procedures; and an opportunity to establish a trusting relationship with one constantly present nurse, who functioned as the child's primary nurse.

☐ Home preparatory materials and stress-point preparation in hospital.

☐ Home preparatory materials and consistent supportive care from a single nurse in the hospital.

☐ Routine nursing care only.

The outcome measures included:

1. Observer rating of the child's level of upset and co-operation during six stress points during the admission.

2. Time to the first urination postoperatively.
3. Post-hospital adjustment, assessed through a parents' questionnaire completed one week after discharge.

The results indicated that all three of the home preparation conditions were significantly better on most of the children's measures than the control condition of routine nursing care. There was no significant difference between any of the preparatory methods. When home preparation was compared to the control condition, there was no improvement in parents' anxiety or satisfaction with care, but improved parental satisfaction occurred when home preparation was followed by stress-point preparation in the hospital, or with consistent supportive care.

In another study, 58 children between the ages of four and seventeen were shown either a hospital-relevant slide–tape information package, or an unrelated film on the night before surgery. A multidimensional assessment battery was used that included a subjective report, behavioural measures, physiological measures, parental report, and operating and recovery room indices. The results indicated that the hospital-relevant information improved the children's experience and recovery from surgery, but age and previous experience affected the amount of information required. Children under the age of eight, and those who had had at least one previous surgery experience were at risk of becoming sensitized by viewing the preparatory material and, in general, had poorer adjustment to the hospital experience (Melamed *et al.*, 1987).

Activity
When you are on a children's ward find out from the Sister what is the ward policy for the psychological preparation of children for invasive procedures or surgery. Who talks to the child? Is it planned and allocated as part of the nursing plan? Is it forgotten if the ward is under pressure? Does the ward consider this aspect is well managed?

The child's consent for medical procedures

The recent trend towards emphasizing and identifying children's rights is affecting nursing practice. Children are being told at school and at home to respect their bodies and are being given some responsibility for themselves, and are learning not to be dominated by adult demands. It is possible that in the future children may have similar rights of consent as adults.

The Department of Health Report (1991) states:

The rights of children to give consent to treatment were reinforced by a judgement in the House of Lords in 1985 [the Gillick case] which stated that 'the parental right to determine whether or not their minor child below the age of 16 years will have medical treatment terminates if and when the child achieves sufficient understanding and intelligence to enable him or her to fully understand what is proposed.'

It follows that young people should be kept as fully informed as possible about their condition and treatment to enable them to exercise their rights. Even where younger children do not have the required understanding they should be provided with as much information as possible and their wishes ascertained and taken into account. A guide to consent for examination and treatment was published by the NHS Executive in 1990.

It is likely that children will gradually become more involved in the process of treatment, and will be treated as independent, thinking individuals, rather than as recipients of a service who should behave and do as they are told. Adults are often unaware of the sophistication and depth of the child's understanding. Talking over the child's bed about the child's condition is a common example of adults' ignorance about child development. Gradually adults are coming to realize their mistake, and junior medical staff and nurses are now warned about talking in front of children.

Consent raises similar questions. The difficulty lies in ascertaining when the child can be considered to be able to give informed consent. Many people still think it impossible for a child to be able to understand bodily functions and medical treatment. Implicit in the issue of preparation is the expectation that if the child understands the process, then they are also giving consent. Information can be presented simply, so that children can understand in ways appropriate to their developmental level. Many adults only have a vague notion of how their bodies work and the effect of medical treatment – even less than some children – but they are still considered able to give consent.

Once consent to treatment has been given, the issue becomes one of how to help the child to cope with the stress of the event, rather than one of imposing procedures on a struggling child. Children can be overwhelmed by the same feelings and anxieties as any adult, and the responsibility lies with the medical and nursing staff to help them to cope in the best way possible, rather than the child carrying the blame for misbehaving. Techniques of helping children to cope with pain and anxiety then become important, and the child is recognized as having skills that can be developed to cope with these situations.

Anxiety and pain management

The psychological management of pain involves helping children to control their perception and expression of pain. The management of pain is a difficult and complex area, but it is clear that anxiety can exacerbate the pain. It is therefore important to reduce the child's level of anxiety in order to reduce the pain and reduce reliance on medication.

The experience of pain occurs in many different conditions. It can be due to a disease state; a physical injury; psychosomatic pain; or pain from medical procedures. The experience of pain also depends on its frequency, severity and duration, as well as how much control the child has over the pain.

Research studies have demonstrated that the development of the concept of pain parallels the evolving concepts of health and illness. Gaffney and Dunn (1986) gave 680 children aged five to fourteen a sentence-completion task relating to various aspects of pain. They proposed that there are three stages in defining the concept of pain:

- concrete definitions of pain, defined by location, e.g. 'a thing in your tummy' (5–7 years);
- semi-abstract definitions of pain, using terms like 'a sore feeling' (8–10 years);
- abstract definitions of pain, e.g., physiological cause and psychological consequences of worry and depression (11+ years).

The measurement of pain may be an issue in the continuing care of some children, particularly those with chronic or recurrent pain and a number of assessment tools are available. The 'Oucher' (Beyer and Aradine, 1986) is comprised of six photographs of a child's face with expressions ranging from neutrality to severe distress, alongside a scale that ranges 0–100. Children can indicate a point on the scale or choose a picture of a face to match the pain they are experiencing.

The child's assessment of their pain can be a valuable guideline for intervention and pain-control strategies. There are different techniques that can be taught to children to help them to cope with pain and to reduce their level of distress. This is called the self-regulation of pain.

Guided imagery

Here the child is helped to think of a pleasant and enjoyable experience they have had, for example, playing on the beach, going to a party, or playing in the garden with their dog. The child is encouraged to imagine the scene and describe details to an adult. Once they can imagine the scene quickly and easily, they can think of it when they are experiencing pain, and distract themselves from thinking about their pain. The imagery is often relaxing and helps to relieve anxiety.

Sometimes the guided imagery a child uses can be specifically orientated towards images that are incompatible with pain. If vasodilation reduces the experience of pain, then images of a hot, sunny day or lying in a warm bath can have an additional effect over and above the distraction and relaxation produced by the imagery. This is often used in biofeedback techniques, where the child is taught to control their autonomic functions by watching visual feedback of their physiological responses.

Relaxation

In progressive muscle relaxation, children learn to tense and relax different muscle groups in the body. Before the age of seven, images of becoming floppy like a rag doll are helpful in explaining to the child the desired physical state. If the child can learn to relax when they are in pain, particularly chronic pain, they can reduce the anxiety and tension associated with the experience of pain. Taking deep breaths through the nose and blowing out in small puffs through the mouth in order to relax is also beneficial.

Hypnotherapy

Hypnosis or self-hypnosis techniques have been used with children suffering pain in a wide variety of acute and chronic conditions. The hypnotic state is induced by encouraging the child to look at one point for a prolonged period, or to concentrate on one part of their arm that is being stroked repeatedly. Selective focusing of attention is used to guide the child's imagination, encouraging relaxation and a sense of well-being and control. Children seem to be able to be hypnotized relatively easily compared with adults. Suggestions of relaxation are made in the context of a simple story, for example, of walking down steps to a warm, comfortable room where they feel happy and have no pain. Sometimes the child's favourite television hero or pop star can be included to help make the pain disappear. Suggestions are made during the relaxed state that will continue post-hypnotically. The child's attention is then brought back to the room where he or she is. Children can rapidly learn to hypnotize themselves using certain words and images, and can use this whenever they feel pain, or are undergoing unpleasant procedures (Olness and Gardner, 1988).

Distraction

This is a technique commonly used by nurses and parents when children are in pain. Encouraging the child to look at a picture, or to watch a balloon, are ways of removing attention from the painful procedure. This may work for children who try to avoid thinking about the pain, but for the actively coping child it may cause irritation as it stops them from concentrating and controlling their own reactions.

Suggestion of pain relief

Gently talking the child through their pain and helping them to think it away is the purpose of this technique. Telling and reassuring the child that the pain is going away has to be tuned into the child's perception of pain; it should not just be a throwaway statement. Helping them to rate the intensity of the pain on a scale, and then encouraging them to reduce the rating down the scale or turn down their pain switch can also help.

The type of coping strategy used will vary from child to child. Some prefer to use distracting methods in order to avoid the pain, while others seek out information in order to cope better and gain control of themselves and the pain. Most children use a range of different methods depending on the situation, who they are with, how severe the pain is, how old they are, and how frightened they are.

Distracting methods include:

- using external events to divert the child's attention from the pain;
- using internal events: the child diverts their attention by concentrating on other feelings in their body;
- using imagery or thinking about other events;
- re-interpreting sensations so the child thinks the sensation is different, e.g., pain is coldness;
- using fantasy, for example, when the child imagines he or she is someone who does not feel pain, or that magic stops them from feeling pain.

Information-seeking and controlling methods include:

- questioning what is happening;
- positive self-statements: children tell themselves they can cope and they are doing well;
- relaxation to feel calm;
- asking for physical help or emotional support and comfort from parents or nurses;
- using an emotional response like crying or screaming to release tension, or inhibiting emotional expression in order to keep control.

Some children who have chronic pain or who are very frightened by acute pain can become difficult to handle. It can be useful for nurses to watch carefully what happens when the child shows distress: it may be that the extreme expression of pain is linked to environmental events and the responses of adults. Children can gain additional sympathy and attention for their distress, which sometimes can make it worse. There is always the concern that reducing the child's expression of pain may lead to the child sitting in pain and not complaining. This is unlikely if the child receives sensitive and individual support in dealing with their pain.

Sometimes a package of different skills is necessary. Elliott and Olson (1983) evaluated a treatment package for reducing the distress of burnt children undergoing stressful procedures of unwrapping bandages, the first 15 minutes of hydrotherapy, and re-wrapping of the burnt areas. The package included attention distraction, relaxation breathing, the use of imagery, re-interpretation of the context of pain, and reinforcement for using the coping techniques. While the children were able to significantly reduce their levels of distress when actively supported by the clinician, it is not clear which components were most effective. It may be that the use of a range of techniques allowed the children to switch between them if one became less effective.

Jay *et al.* (1985) also used a package of techniques with five children aged three to seven with leukaemia to reduce the anxiety and distress associated with bone marrow aspirations and lumbar punctures. The intervention included:

- Breathing exercises, using imagery as an attention-distraction procedure.
- Reinforcement in the form of a trophy for lying still and doing the breathing exercises.
- Imagery, using heroic images to change the context of pain.
- Behavioural rehearsal where the child and a staff member use dolls to role-play treatment procedures. This includes desensitization to reduce fear, and information-giving and modelling so the child can observe what will happen.
- Filmed modelling, which described a six-year-old coping with a bone marrow aspiration and a spinal tap.

All of the children showed a reduction in distress as measured on the Observation Scale of Behavioural Distress, and no child required restraint during the procedures.

Pain management in emergencies

In emergencies there is no time for preparation and rehearsal. Olness (1989) has commented that more than 80% of children over the age of two may benefit from hypnotherapy strategies used in accident and emergency settings, even though the children have had no previous experience of hypnosis. Olness has outlined a procedure for nurses to help children in emergency situations:

➤ **Be positive in statements to the child**. Staff's reactions and statements if they are negative – 'That's a bad cut', 'What a terrible bruise' – can undermine the child's attempts to cope with pain. Positive comments should be made to the child about his or her physical state, e.g., 'Your blood looks good and strong', 'We are going to sew that cut up to make it heal faster.' Nurses should say they are there to help the child to get better. Positive suggestions that the treatment will make the pain get better can help the child reassess the situation; washing a wound helps to 'wash' away the pain if the child is encouraged to relax and 'go floppy' while being treated.

➤ **Enhance the child's sense of mastery**. The aim should always be to enhance the child's ability to cope by telling him or her what is happening and what is going to happen next. Explaining where they are going, what the noises are, and who you are, helps to make sense of the new and frightening surroundings. The child should be given permission to scream in order to gain control, 'You can cry if you want to but I shall be here holding your hand'; asking the child to scream louder will demonstrate to the child that he or she has some control.

➤ **Make personal contact with the child**. If there is a little time, the nurse can find out something about the child. 'What do you like doing best?', 'Do you have any favourite pop stars, football teams, television programmes, hobbies?', etc. If the child will not talk, then making statements and guesses about how he or she is feeling can be a way of gaining acknowledgement.

Summary

Good psychological care of children in hospital has been demonstrated to have a positive effect on the child's health and speed of recovery. Poor psychological care can disturb and upset the child's emotional and behavioural development over a long period after leaving hospital. In treating and caring for the whole child's needs, the nurse's aims therefore should be to provide the best emotionally supportive environment for the child whilst in hospital.

This commences on the child's admission to hospital and includes the involvement of the family in the care and support of the child throughout the admission. Nurses need to be aware of the parents' needs as well as the child's in order to support them throughout their ordeal. Children of differing ages will raise issues specific to their age groups and nurses should be aware of the needs of adolescents in particular. Play and education are of significant importance for all hospitalized children and provision should be made for this.

Children experience a number of unpleasant and invasive procedures while in hospital and they should receive preparation appropriate to their needs and preferences. Some children are active copers with these stresses while others are avoidant. Nurses should realize that children have equal rights and needs as adults to full information, appropriate to their developmental level, about procedures they are to undergo.

Developing a sensitive and trusting relationship with the child and parents is essential to enable the child to cope with the unpleasant experiences. The nurse will then become sensitized to the pain control needs of children and aid them in finding methods of pain control that are most effective.

7 Care of the dying child

Introduction

Death is a distressing topic for most of us. We try to put it out of our minds, and it rarely confronts us in everyday life. We do not like to think of our own death, and our direct experience of it may be limited to the loss of a pet. Only some nurses will have a personal understanding of the feelings of loss, guilt, and anger that accompany the finality of death.

The death of a child is a particularly distressing event as it raises a range of feelings about lost hope, lost expectations, a lost future, and the loss of the child's faith in the parents' or the doctors' ability to protect and save them.

Dying and death at whatever age can be peaceful and harmonious or agonizing and distressing for all concerned. Nurses caring for a dying child can enable and facilitate the inevitable process in a comforting and safe way, so that the parents and the child feel supported, contained, and understood.

The child's understanding of death

In order to be able to talk to children about death and answer their questions, health professionals should be aware of how much the child understands about the concept itself. Children as young as three know that death occurs, but they may not grasp the full implications until they are past eight. Those children who have had some experience of death, or who have talked about it, often have a more advanced concept than other children. Adolescents usually have an adult concept of what death means.

The idea of death includes several components that together bring about a full understanding of what it means. Children will have a grasp of some, but not necessarily all, of these. Kane (1979) suggests that the following contribute to understanding the concept of death:

Realization (understood by most three-year-olds)

Even very young children have an awareness of death.

Separation (understood by most five-year-olds)

Young children can be very aware that death means separation from their parents, friends, or brothers and sisters. This may be their main concept, and they may be concerned that they will feel lonely, or that their parents will be lonely without them.

Immobility (understood by most five-year-olds)

The awareness that dead people cannot move can concern some children, who are not also aware that dead people cannot feel, see, or hear.

Irrevocability (understood by most six-year-olds)

The fact that once people die they cannot come back to life again is essential in understanding death. Many children younger than five or six may not realize the finality of the process. Children play games at being shot and dying, but then leap to life the next minute. 'Pretend' death and 'real' death need to be made clear, so that the child realizes that 'real' death means never living again.

Causality (understood by most six-year-olds)

There is always a physical cause of death. Young children, however, often have magical ideas about what causes death, for example a nasty wish, saying something horrible, or being naughty can sometimes be perceived as having caused illness or death. Children need to understand that it is not such imaginary events that cause death, but that something is wrong with their body which is causing them to die.

Dysfunctionality (understood by most six-year-olds)

Explanations about death to children should include the cessation of bodily functions, for example, that the body stops breathing, growing, seeing, hearing, thinking, and feeling, and the heart stops beating. Some children worry they might be able to hear when they are dead but not be able to tell anyone.

Universality (understood by most eight-year-olds)

That every living organism dies at some time is important in understanding that everyone must eventually die. This idea can comfort some children, who may believe that everyone lives for ever, and that it is unfair that they are dying.

Insensitivity (understood by most eight-year-olds)

That a dead person cannot feel anything is often difficult for young children to understand. For example, if they walk on a grave, they may wonder if they are 'hurting' the person under the ground. One way of helping a child who is dying in pain, or who has experienced pain during their illness or treatment is to help them to realize they will never feel pain again after death, which can perhaps be a welcome relief for children who have suffered a lot. They may even express a wish to die in order to escape the pain and distress they feel.

Appearance (understood by most twelve-year-olds)

A dead body looks different to a living body, and children may be very interested in the physical characteristics of death. They can seem ghoulish sometimes in their desire for detailed descriptions of what a dead person looks like.

The difficulty with assessing children's knowledge of the concept of death is the dependence on verbal expression. Lansdown and Benjamin (1985) found that children who are more verbally competent have a more complete concept of death. It may be that children are aware of the concept of death before they are able to express it adequately.

It is only by talking with children about death that nurses can understand how much they know. Brief comments from a child may reveal surprising misunderstandings, or a sophisticated view. Young children sometimes appear to have a well-developed notion of death, but when this is examined more closely it may only apply to old people and not to children – and certainly not to themselves. When children were asked, 'Do you believe that some day you will die?', the following percentage said 'yes': age five, 50%; age six, 73%; age seven, 82%; ages eight to ten, 100% (Reilly *et al.*, 1983). Lansdown (1989) outlined stages in the concept of illness that contribute to an awareness of death:

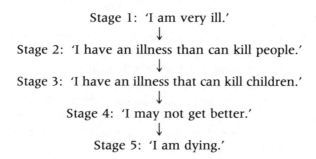

Stage 1: 'I am very ill.'
↓
Stage 2: 'I have an illness than can kill people.'
↓
Stage 3: 'I have an illness that can kill children.'
↓
Stage 4: 'I may not get better.'
↓
Stage 5: 'I am dying.'

Stage 3 is the critical realization that the child's illness can kill other children. Children of different ages will have passed through different stages, and it is important to understand what the child is thinking about him or herself, as well as their more abstract thoughts of what death means.

Exercise

Which concepts of death are the following statements demonstrating?

- 'Jesus will make me better with kisses and send me back.'
- 'Children can die of no food or crossing the road.'
- 'She can't get out of the graveyard because they lock the box, don't they?'
- 'Does it hurt him if I stand on his grave?'
- 'Toys don't die. They last forever, but we don't.'
- 'I'll be lonely without you in heaven.'

Communicating with dying children

One of the most important aspects of nursing the dying child is to take the time to provide the necessary attention when the child wants to talk about their illness or the future. Sometimes questions are direct and to the point, for example, 'Am I going to die?'; others may be indirect, for example, 'Why am I having my birthday presents now when my birthday isn't until next month?' It is essential that the nurse is prepared for such questions, and is able to know what approach to take.

Nurses need to know the attitudes and the policy of each ward. If it is the policy that only senior nursing staff or doctors talk to children and families about prognosis and death, then nurses need to know how to divert a child's potentially distressing question without upsetting him or her. There should be a method of indicating to colleagues that the question has been asked, and that the child needs to understand what is happening. Some medical staff feel the parents are the best people to talk to their child.

A child who is questioning and indicating that they know they might be dying should have their queries answered clearly and openly. They may be having upsetting fantasies about death, and talking about it will often allow such fantasies to be expressed and the child to be helped. A child kept in secrecy can feel alone and abandoned by the people they have learned to trust, at a time when they are most vulnerable. Children are sensitive to non-verbal signals, tones of voice, and expressions from staff and family members: they see their parents crying, or they detect a change in the parent's relationship and feelings towards them. Some parents become closer and more involved once warned of impending death; others may withdraw and try to conceal their feelings. These lines from a poem written by a dying child to her mother (quoted in Mulholland, 1973), summarize succinctly the child's need for information:

> 'Worst of all was the agony
> Of not knowing
> What you knew.'

The general view at present is that the parents' wishes should be respected regarding whether the child should be told that he or she is dying. Most nursing staff, however, would try to persuade reluctant parents to talk about these issues, or request permission to talk with the child about what is going to happen. It is a difficult situation when parents refuse to talk openly with their dying child, as staff are aware the child is asking for information. Whose rights are paramount, the parents' or the child's? The parents may be unable to face the reality that their child is dying, and so will not talk about it, even though it is obvious. Their reluctance to talk to their child is often based in their own inability to cope. Although some parents need to deny the reality of their child's impending death in order to survive emotionally, it is important that this is not imposed on the child. If the parents can permit health professionals to talk with their child about the topics that they cannot face, they are recognizing their child has separate needs from their own, which should be met.

A dying child is often far more able to cope with the information of their death than their parents. Once told about their death, many a young child has shown a far greater awareness and empathy for their parents' feelings than many parents can show their child, because they cannot bear to contemplate death. The child accepts it and does not have hysterics or fall into a deep depression, as might be expected. They may be sad and upset about the thought of leaving their family and pets or not going back to school, but with the support of a loving and caring family, the child's last months and weeks can be calm and accepting of the inevitability of death.

Unfortunately, many children detect that death should not be mentioned. They may worry that it will upset their parents too much if they talk about it, and so they remain quiet in order to protect their family. This becomes an additional burden for the child, on top of coping with their illness and treatments. Just because a child is not asking questions does not mean they are not thinking. They may see the deaths of other children on the ward, or they may know of other children with the same condition who have died. Some children become withdrawn or moody, or start to show difficult behaviour if they cannot talk about such things. When eventually the issue of death and dying is raised, the child may feel a great sense of relief that it has come out into the open, and they can then share their thoughts and anxieties. For some children, just knowing they are going to die is enough to make them relax and understand what is happening; others may ask more questions and start to explore their concerns about what death means.

Children often select who they want to talk to about death and dying. It may be another child, a sibling, a particular nurse, teacher, or playleader. If there is a policy of openness towards the child's questions, it is easier for everyone to feel more relaxed in talking with the child about illness and death.

Knowing what to say

Talking to a dying child can be very difficult. Sharing colleagues' and senior nursing staff's experiences, how they have managed in similar situations and the types of expressions and phrases they have used, can be helpful.

The nurse should find out from the child what they already know, what they think or suspect, and what they really want to know. As Elisabeth Kübler-Ross (1983) says, 'Although all patients have the right to know, not all patients have the need to know.' The child should then be allowed to share his or her worries and have the opportunity to ask questions.

Reflecting a child's questions back to them is an effective way of encouraging the expression of feelings. For example, if a child suddenly asks, 'Am I going to die?', the response could be, 'Do you think you are going to die:', or, 'What makes you think you are going to die?' They may show a good understanding about the severity of their illness, or they may just say they think so because they saw mummy crying. This provides a lead to what is worrying them; they may not actually be asking about death, but about why their parents are so upset.

Questions about death might occur in the context of discussions about their illness and treatments. This is often a useful point at which to answer questions openly, for example the nurse can say, 'You do have an illness that makes some children die but mummy and daddy and we all hope that you won't die.' If the prognosis is poor and active treatment has stopped, then openness and clarity about the future should be addressed simply and clearly. Planning ahead for this eventuality is necessary so that all ward staff and the child's parents know what has been said, and by whom.

Some children ask questions about death suddenly and unexpectedly.

They may blurt out a worry that has been on their mind for some time, or an event may trigger off the thought, for example, when they realize that another child on the ward has died. This may be the first time the question has been asked, or the child may have already asked five people since morning. If a child does not understand the answer, or does not get the answer they need, they will repeatedly ask the question.

Other children make comments or indirect statements that indicate their concerns and challenge a response, for example, 'I don't suppose I'll be here for my birthday', or, 'There's no point in making Christmas decorations'. Both indicate the child's awareness but inability to ask the direct question. If such queries are fended off with bland reassurances, the child will not be helped to express concerns, and may not make any further attempts to find out what is happening.

If treatment has stopped, or a child is very ill and is going to die and yet the issue of death has not been raised by the child, it will be necessary to discuss with the parents how to raise it. Some children may not have even thought of it; others may be worrying deep inside and yet feel unable to ask anyone. It is often helpful to allow the possibility of questions to be raised while doing an activity, for example, talking while doing a craft activity or drawing is one way of being close and talking with a child about the difficult topic of their condition.

Enquiring about the child's previous experience of death can be another way into the discussion. If a pet or a relative has died, this can introduce the topic in a distant way. Enquiring about the child's feelings at the time, their knowledge about what happened, and what was said to them can lead to talking about different beliefs and explanations about death. If the child wants to ask questions, it should be made clear that all queries will be answered as simply and directly as possible.

The dying adolescent

Whether healthy or ill, adolescents are in the ambiguous position of being neither adults nor children. Many will have the understanding of an adult about the concept of death, but will experience conflict regarding the future. Adams and Deveau (1986) have identified a range of common responses to adolescents' knowledge of their own impending death:

Denial

Denial is part of the process of trying to understand what is happening.

It can be a dynamic process that is subject to change depending on new information or mood, and it can be a positive or a negative reaction. Denial can allow the adolescent time to absorb little pieces of information over time while carrying on living. But it can be negative if it is rigid and entrenched.

Anger

This can result in rebellion and non-cooperation. Anger can be expressed towards staff or parents, the surroundings and routines in the hospital, or the treatment procedures.

Anxiety

Apart from the anxiety generated by the illness and the treatments, the adolescent can start to worry about the meaning of death.

Sadness and depression

Sadness and depression are part of dying and adolescents will move in and out of phases of depression. A complete clinical depression is not common.

Guilt

Guilt may prevent an adolescent from expressing his or her feelings, or from seeking the help that they require. Cultural or family influences may instil these feelings, which are very difficult to resolve. If parents are unable to accept the reality of their dying child, they may impose covert restrictions on the adolescent discussing it, for fear of hurting them.

Withdrawal

This is one of the most common responses. It allows the adolescent time to escape from an anxiety-provoking situation, and provides time for them to regain their strength and confront what lies ahead.

Over-compensation

The determination to achieve high goals provides adolescents with a channel for their energy, and directs them away from anxiety and death. They may set themselves physical, intellectual, or creative goals that need to be achieved before they die.

Regression

If they feel overwhelmed by their illness they may revert to an earlier stage of development. This is often precipitated by severe physical or emotional stress, and parents may need help in understanding what is happening. For example, an adolescent who seemed independent and striving for control may become dependent and immature in their behaviour and emotional state.

Adams and Deveau (1986) have outlined specific guidelines to nursing staff caring for dying adolescents:

- Facilitate access to parents and special health team members.
- Keep the nursing staff as constant as possible, and narrow down the total number of staff involved in providing care.
- Allow the adolescent a continuing role in decision making. Involve the parents and the adolescent in discussions about the right to refuse treatment or resuscitation; encourage the participation of siblings.
- Provide the patient with time alone to rest, free from interruptions. Recognize the distancing from staff and family as a natural phenomenon.
- Provide opportunities for parents to comfort their adolescents by hand-holding, gentle stroking, rubbing, washing, and so on.
- Give pain medication without hesitation, and make sure it is effective.
- Provide nursing measures like warm baths, gentle rubs, quiet music.

Talking to the parents of a dying child

When a child is terminally ill, there is often time to gradually help parents come to realize that their child is going to die. This can occur over a period of time, during which the child will have received extensive treatment and prognosis. The results of the treatment will have been discussed repeatedly with medical staff, and the parents will sometimes be able to see for themselves there is no further hope.

Because some parents feel inhibited when talking with doctors and are unable to ask questions, the nurse is often the person to whom they turn to express their worries and concerns. The nurse may be the first person to be asked about the long term prospects for their child. They may ask for an opinion about whether their child is going to die. Events on the ward and the deaths of other children with the same illness may all heighten the parents' awareness of the possibility of their own child's death. In other instances, the child's questions may have prompted them suddenly to think of death. When the topic of death arises voluntarily, the nurse can take the opportunity to help the parents to air the possibilities. Most often, they do not want a detailed analysis of the probabilities of survival, or even any involved information about the course of the child's illness – they just want to share their feelings. They need to hear that it is possible that their child could die, although everything possible is being done to avoid that outcome.

When it has been made clear by medical staff that nothing further can be done for the child, then both the nurse and the parents move on to a new stage of coping with the child's illness. Unfortunately, some doctors find this a very difficult statement to make, or may not realize themselves that the child is going to die. If this occurs, it is not possible for the families and nursing staff to move on to the next stage. Preparing for the child's death is prevented, and remains unacknowledged.

Medical treatment always fosters the hope that the child will be cured, so it can be a great shock to parents when they realize that nothing further can be done for their child. They may deny this, and fight against giving up hope. Although medical and nursing staff do not want to make them hopeless, it is important that parents realize the truth of the situation so that they can start to come to terms with what is going to happen, and help their child as much as possible. The strength of the nursing relationship can be crucial during this period. Parents need time and repeated opportunities to discuss what is happening and to share their views and worries with nursing staff. For nurses to sit and listen to the parents while they express their grief or denial is essential if the parents are to come to terms with the agony of what is happening. It is important that the nurses do not try to make the pain go away or to speed up the process of adaptation; it is vital that they are not drawn into 'making things better'. Statements that try to help cushion the distress like, 'Perhaps he will be better off in the long run' (when a child is in severe pain) or 'You can always have another child' may completely miss the feelings the parents are experiencing and denies the reality of their special relationship with the child. Nurses should not impose their own views on parents. This is the time for the parents to work out their own feelings in a safe and supportive environment.

Farewells and endings

In families where the child's death has been anticipated, as death draws nearer the child and the parents need to have the opportunity to say goodbye and to complete any final tasks. As adults make wills to bequeath their possessions, so some children may benefit from thinking about this. Kuykendall (1989) describes how a six-year-old dying of leukaemia decided he wanted to give away his collection of baseball caps to his siblings and friends. He made a list of how many were to go to each person, which was his way of saying goodbye and completing any unfinished business. If parents or staff try to stop this process, thinking it is morbid preoccupation, the child will be denied the opportunity to say goodbye in the way he or she needs to.

The child may want to return home for a last time to say goodbye to their house and toys, or they may request certain toys and possessions to be brought to the hospital. The extended family may collect to say goodbye in turns. The child may want to draw a special picture for classmates to remember them by. The nurse can facilitate this process by asking the child if there is anything they feel they still need to do, and whether they need any help. The requests may be painful for the parents and nursing staff to hear, but by acknowledging the request, reality is also acknowledged. The child and the parents need time for farewells, which can be direct or symbolic.

Where should the child die?

Once staff and family have acknowledged the impending death, preparations and decisions can be made about how to best care for the child and family. A busy acute ward in hospital is not the place for the type of support that is now needed, and the process of waiting for a child to die does not mix easily with the ethos of a ward geared to treatment and discharge. Most acute wards would find long-term care of a dying child difficult and inappropriate.

Once the decision has been made that a child is no longer to receive active medical treatment, and is to be supported only on medication to ease any pain, the possibility of the child going home is usually raised. Sometimes this is brought up before parents are able to accept the finality of the situation, and they may be unable to make decisions and plans to take the child home. Most parents, however, prefer to have their child at home in familiar surroundings for as long as possible during the terminal stages.

Extensive liaison with community services is needed to help the parents feel supported away from the hospital. This is particularly important for families who have become dependent on the hospital during a long and drawn out treatment programme. If they are sent home after many months, or even years, of treatment, they may feel abandoned and left to cope with the death on their own. Some hospitals have ward–home liaison teams, which provide continued care in the community, suppporting the family and community health care staff with information, equipment, and care details for the family and child (Lauer and Camitta, 1980).

Many families find that having their dying child at home is a time of coming to terms with the impending death. The parents have more time to see each other and to talk to each other, rather than visiting, or staying in, hospital. They can take time to express their feelings together. The child sees more of their family and friends; siblings have a greater opportunity to be with their ill brother or sister, and to acknowledge what is happening. The dying child often feels greater comfort and confidence that they will not be alone or with a stranger when they die. In cancer patients, this is often a time of remission of symptoms; the child appears and feels well, and so can take advantage of special treats and attention.

Other parents decide they require more help during the final few weeks or days, when the child needs increased medication for symptom control. Sometimes they want to return to the safety of the hospital ward, where the child was well known; other families prefer a hospice. The development of the hospice movement has been of great benefit to parents and children, providing a medical setting during the terminal stages. The staff are ready and able to cope with the pain and grief of death, and are able to provide a supportive and empathic environment where the needs of the child and family are fully met (Dominica, 1987).

The death of a child in hospital

Intensive care wards and oncology wards experience the most children's deaths and develop their own methods of coping with the stress. Admission to an intensive care ward can mean the child's life will be preserved for a relatively long period with high technology equipment, extensive monitoring, and special care. It can also mean that a child or baby is admitted suddenly and dies within a few hours or a few days, before nursing staff have had time to get to know the child or the family. Each of these circumstances creates a different level of involvement for nurses. It is difficult for health professionals to feel a high level of empathy for a family and child who are hardly known to them, while the fight for life with another family may involve nurses totally and be extremely distressing.

If deaths are part of the ward experience, it is important for there to be a supportive environment to cope with the families' as well as the staffs' reactions. There should be formal and informal recognition of the need for emotional support, which should be part of the running of the ward. Time for this should be scheduled in to the daily and weekly organization of ward life, as well as recognition of the need for flexibility at times of crisis.

Someone needs to take responsibility for informing members of staff who may be off duty of an imminent or actual death of a child, so that they have the opportunity to visit if they want to, or are prepared for the empty bed when they walk on to the ward the next day. Good communication and recognition of others' feelings are essential.

It is also important for the family to have one or two nursing staff with whom they have special contact at the time of death so that their wishes and needs are managed. This can be a difficult role for a nurse if the child's death is sudden or rapid. Parents may be in shock, not able to realize what is happening, and the whole process of preparation and discussion is curtailed into a short period of crisis.

Religious differences and varying patterns of mourning and grief reaction all have to be acknowledged and understood. Due to their religious beliefs, parents may be greatly offended and upset by inappropriate management of the body after death and so it is important to find out their views, or make sure an interpreter is available to help out with communication. The hospital chaplain will usually have contacts with other religious leaders, and will be able to give advice.

If parents are not staying in the hospital with the child, they must be contacted immediately if there is any likelihood of the child dying. If they are coming in unexpectedly to the ward they will need to feel contained by the staff, and helped to have privacy in order to express their grief together with their child. They will feel confused and shocked, and will have to absorb distressing information quickly.

When the child dies, health professionals should check with the parents whether they prefer company or privacy while with their child. Parents should be encouraged to touch the dead child and cuddle the body if they want to. The removal of the attached lines and equipment will make the child seem more theirs, and they will see him or her uncluttered and peaceful in a way that he or she may not have been seen for days or weeks. Some parents want a photograph of their child to take home, so it is worth asking whether they would like the nurse to arrange this.

It is essential at this stage for parents to feel they have time, and that they are not being hurried so the nurses can prepare the body or arrange the bed for someone else. Some families may need to be told that siblings too can see the dead child if they want to. Often the feelings of siblings are left out at a time like this and it can help the process of grieving and mourning if everyone sees the dead body. Everyone needs a chance to say goodbye, and to say what they wish to the child.

Nurses also need time to talk to the other parents and children on the ward while all of this is happening. The flurry of activity in one cubicle or behind the drawn curtains, staff expressions, and hearing the sounds of grief will upset other families, who will be suddenly reminded of the possibility and imminence of death. They may become more demanding because of their concern, and want to know what is happening. They also need to know what to tell their own ill children.

After the child's death

Once arrangements have been made for the disposal of the child's body, the parents go home alone with their loss. The funeral is often their last visit to the hospital, where they may have spent many months during the child's illness. Ward staff have been involved in the care of the child, and it is important to the families that nurses show concern after death as well as before it. The loss of contact with ward staff and the hospital itself can be an additional loss for the parents whose lives may have been totally occupied with visiting their ill child. A total readjustment has to take place.

In recognition of this, the parents should be encouraged to come back and visit the staff and see where their child died when they feel able and when they want to. If they have not visited within a month after the death, it is useful for the sister or significant nurse to write or telephone the family to ask how they are, enquiring specifically whether they want to come back to visit. Some parents feel shy about visiting unless invited and will feel a great sense of relief that they and their child have not been forgotten. They may benefit greatly from talking about the course of the child's illness and death with nurses who were present at the time. They may raise anxieties and worries they had not previously mentioned, or they may express guilt or fantasies about what could have happened. Talking about the good times in hospital and the funny experiences that occurred are all part of reviewing what happened, and can help parents to feel that positive and fond memories also exist. Small details of memories and experiences that different nurses had with the child are all valuable for parents to hear.

Nurses can help the parents by keeping photographs or small items that belonged to the child until they come to retrieve them, perhaps several months after the death. The time of death may have been too distressing and painful for parents to realize what they wanted to keep, but a later opportunity to have small toys, a name-tag or a little blanket can be precious momentos that are treasured.

Family bereavement and mourning

Bereavement reactions of parents after the loss of a baby or a child vary widely. Initially they may be shocked and unable to recognize what has happened. A high psychiatric morbidity has been associated with neonatal death (White *et al.*, 1984). Poor support is a contributory factor, and half of the parents seen reported psychiatric problems 16 months after the death.

Bereavement counselling in the community after a child's death is not readily available, and so some families benefit from joining a group that will give them support. Nurses can help them to find out what is available locally, or liaise with community nurses to ensure that parents are given the address of CRUSE or any other support groups or counselling help. Forrest *et al.* (1981) compared 25 families receiving counselling with 25 receiving routine hospital care after the death of their baby, and at six months the counselled group were significantly less disturbed. This equalized by 14 months, at which time 80% were symptom-free, yet 20% still had problems.

Bereavement reactions continue for a long time after the death of a child, and many parents wonder if they will ever be able to cope normally again. In severe cases where parents are impeded in their daily living by long-term grief reaction, a technique of directed grief and mourning has had some success. It involves taking the parents through the steps of the loss at their own pace, and may include visits to the burial place, or back to the hospital in order to resurrect the experience and help the parents to progress through their feelings (Mawson, *et al.*, 1981).

Summary

Children's death is a topic that all health professionals need to acknowledge and prepare themselves for. To be able to support and care for dying children and their families, nurses should be sensitive to the child's understanding of what death means so that questions can be answered appropriately for the child's conceptual level.

Communicating with children about death requires openness and information when children ask questions and also requires nurses to be aware of children's non-verbal signals. Nurses may need to raise the topic gently with children who are reluctant to ask about what they already fear. Similarly, parents may require support and encouragement to talk to their child about death.

Health professionals should prepare themselves for children's questions at awkward moments and be ready to acknowledge the questions and use the opportunity to find out about the child's perception and understanding. Dying adolescents show a range of emotional reactions some of which are difficult for nurses to cope with. A withdrawn, angry adolescent will require time and patience from nurses to gradually accept the inevitable.

Children can benefit from the opportunity to formally say goodbye to friends, places and belongings. This can be linked with the child going home to die or having a final period at home before ultimately returning to hospital when the family can no longer cope.

Death may be sudden and unexpected or prolonged and anticipated on hospital wards and so nurses need to be prepared for the different cultural, religious and emotional needs of families. Patterns of grief and mourning will vary and nurses should support parents in saying goodbye to their child in a private and personal way.

After the child's death, parents should be encouraged to return to talk about their child and the final stages of life when they are able to. Parents should not be forgotten after the death of their child. Bereavement counselling may be necessary in the community or at the hospital to help parents acknowledge their loss.

Further reading

Carr, C. and McNeil, J. (1986). *Adolescence and Death*. Springer, New York.
    Provides a view of the specialist needs of adolescents and recognizes the
    range of behaviour and emotional reactions that dying adolescents show.

Landsown, R. and Goldman, A. (1988). The psychological care of children with
    malignant disease. *Journal of Child Psychology and Psychiatry, 29*, 555–567.
    This article provides a review of work with oncology and haematology
    patients. It raises the psychological support required and how the family can
    be involved in treatment including the reactions of siblings. Communicating
    with children and the concept of death and illness are also included.

SECTION THREE

Caring for the carers

8 Be aware of yourself

The effects of stress

Stress may be consciously recognized, or it may demonstrate its effects without the person being fully aware of what is causing the problem. The effects may be physical or psychological. If the stress is chronic, then feelings can start to affect general physical functioning, for example, headaches, sexual difficulties, hypertension, or coronary artery disease. Over the long term, psychological effects can result in states of anxiety or depression, and relationship problems.

Chronic stress that goes unrecognized or unaided can lead to 'burn-out'. Nurses start to lose interest in their jobs, and lack energy, enthusiasm, and commitment to work they previously enjoyed. Sometimes this is accompanied by physical illness. It may lead to exhaustion, susceptibility to illnesses, taking time off work, over-eating, drinking or smoking excessively, and resorting to medication and drugs to aid sleep and relaxation. One study found that burn-out in nurses was correlated with the percentage of children on the unit with social or behavioural problems (Pagel and Wittmann, 1986).

Activity
Identify any symptoms of stress you have experienced in the past. Below are lists of commonly reported psychological and physiological symptoms. Which do you tend to have?

Psychological symptoms	Physiological symptoms
irritability	hyperventilation
forgetfulness	trembling
preoccupation	weakness
poor concentration	cold hands and feet
depressive thoughts	butterflies
anxious thoughts	nausea/vomiting
inability to cope	headaches/migraine
feelings of worthlessness	poor appetite
exhaustion	palpitations
feelings of hopelessness	
poor sleep	

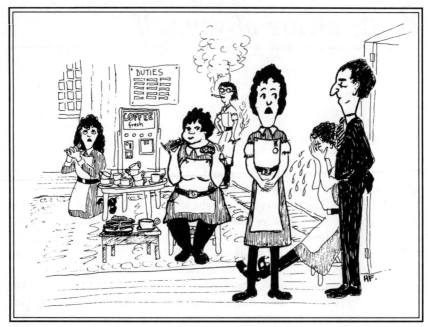

We all have our own way of coping with stress.

The causes of stress

Cox (1978) concludes that there are three major approaches to the study of causes of stress:

1. Stress as a feeling: for example, an individual's response to a stressful situation.
2. Stress as an event or series of events: for example, characteristics of stressful environments.
3. Stress as an experience: for example, a lack of fit between the individual and the environment.

The last classification emphasizes stress as a product of the relationship between human beings and their environment, and focuses on the personal nature of that experience. It takes into account the importance of the individual's reactions to events, and also the stressful events themselves.

People are not passive recipients of stress: any response to stressful events in the environment is affected by personality, perception, and understanding of the stress, as well as previous experiences. Feelings of stress seem to occur when the perceived demands of the situation are not matched by the perceived ability to cope with them (Bailey 1985). The demands may be physical, emotional, or social, and arise in personal or work life experiences. The experience of stress is highly subjective, and is related to each person's perception of the relationship between the cause and the effect of stress, and the way in which the harmful effects can be reduced (Goodwin, 1987).

Douglas (1985) has drawn a useful distinction between sources of stress. Exogenous stress originates from outside the person and includes lack of control and lack of autonomy; endogenous stress originates inside the person and includes the pressure placed upon oneself. Endogenous stress has also been recognized when nurses' expectations are very different to reality, particularly when the student nurse has to compromise his or her ideals with the realities of the work context once they reach the ward.

Sources of stress

Stressful Events	Experienced	Created Stress

Stress in personal life

Personal illness
Bereavement
Illness in relatives or family
Moving house
Housing problems
Financial problems
Changing jobs
Travelling or commuting
   difficulties
Problems with partner
Problems with friends
Problems with relatives

Stress at work

Interpersonal difficulties
Poor communication with
   colleagues
Conflicts of personalities
Feeling undervalued

Organizational stress
Chronic work overload
Role conflict and ambiguity
Policy changes
New organizational structures
Poor management
Conflicting priorities
Low morale

Patient-related stress
Difficult patients and families
Stressful nursing procedures

Sources of stress (continued)

Stressful Events	Experienced	Created Stress
High emotional involvement with patients		
Poor emotional professional support		
Death and dying		
Environmental stress		
Poor physical working conditions		
Poor physical living conditions		
Overcrowding		
Noise		
Heat and cold		

Activity

Can you pinpoint any of these situations that have created stress in your own life? Now try to identify why you experienced stress in these situations. Has it been created by the events, or by your personal reaction to the events? Would everyone have reacted in the way you did? For example, you may have moved accommodation several times and enjoyed the process of change and the challenge of finding a new place, or you may have experienced a lot of worry and disturbance because you do not like change – or both.

You may realize that the list omits the personal dimension of how and why you react to an event. This demonstrates how stress questionnaires that focus on the environment alone will produce varying results according to the individual who fills them in.

Studies have identified particular stressors for health professionals, including heavy workload, high responsibility, insufficient time to work or to relax, frequent experiences of emotional and physical exhaustion, and fatigue. For nursing staff, the following have been highlighted: poor working conditions, staff shortages, high responsibility with minimal authority, and poor pay.

In a study of staff stress in a children's hospice Woolley *et al.* (1989) used interviews, scores on the General Health Questionnaire, rate of sick leave, staff turnover, and ratings of job satisfaction to assess the level of staff stress experienced. They found that 25% of the staff showed significant signs of stress. The main symptoms were anxiety, insomnia, some somatic symptoms, and social dysfunction.

The highest levels of stress were created by nursing children with uncontrollable symptoms, and witnessing children in pain and mental distress. Staff indicated that their ability to relieve symptoms or distress was rewarding in their work. Forty-two per cent of the staff found it difficult to cope with the negative responses of families, particularly expressions of anger, helplessness, and criticism. Patients who did not show signs of grieving left staff feeling uncertain about how to relate to and support them.

Eighty per cent of the staff found that difficulties in staff communication and interrelationships were an important source of stress. All of the staff felt that informal staff support was the most important factor in helping them to cope. Other factors included having a sense of humour; knowing their own limitations and skills; having a philosophy that helped them through the bad times; and support from friends and relatives. The implications that arose for selection and support of staff were important. Staff that experienced the most stress had either suffered a past bereavement or were experiencing one currently.

Lattanzi (1985) identified the sense of powerlessness associated with being unable to save a dying child, or to eliminate the pain of bereavement. It is important that staff do not feel diminished by a sense of helplessness while nursing dying children. Even on highly specialized units there is little agreement about the primary sources of stress for nursing staff. Keane *et al.* (1985) found no indication that ICU nurses could be differentiated from non-ICU nurses on measures of state/trait anxiety, negative self-concepts, feelings of hopelessness, entrapment, or frustration. Another study reported that levels of job satisfaction and morale were higher among ICU nurses than those on renal, medical, and surgical wards (Nichols *et al.*, 1981).

Hipwell *et al.* (1989) took a socio-psychological perspective by identifying the causes of stress on a coronary care unit, a renal unit, a general medical ward, and an acute geriatric ward, and related these to the nurses' perceptions of the social climate of their work environments. They found that the average stress scores for the four wards were very similar. Death, dying, and work load were identified as the most important stressors for all the nurses. The non-specialized nurses generally experienced slightly more stress than the specialized nurses.

Another questionnaire that has been used consists of 30 items subdivided into subscales assessing the five major sources of job stress among nurses. It has been used to assess stress in nursing managers as well as nurses in high-risk jobs like intensive care and hospice nursing (Cooper and Mitchell, 1990). The scale includes:

➤ Managing workload: the pressure due to feelings of insufficient time and resources to complete tasks and meet deadlines.
➤ Organizational support and involvement: the perceived pressure of lack of involvement in planning and decision-making at work, and issues about inadequate feedback.
➤ Dealing with patients and relatives: the patients' relationship with the nurse, and the nurse's feelings about death and dying.

➤ Home/work conflict.
➤ Confidence and competence: the difficulties experienced with the nursing role, and the problems of coping with change and responsibility.

Coping with stress

People cope with stress in very different ways. One theory sees stress as a relationship between the person and the environment, where stress is appraised as exceeding the person's resources and endangering well-being.

Coping involves thinking about and doing activities to reduce the impact of stress. Two processes are considered to mediate stressful experiences: primary appraisal is the process of perceiving a personal threat, that is, events seen as irrelevant, benign, or harmful; secondary appraisal occurs when individuals evaluate the adequacy of their resources to prevent harm to themselves and to organize a potential response. Coping is the carrying out of this response in order to alleviate distress, or to aid in dealing with the problem causing the distress. This action becomes a buffer that moderates the impact of stress. Lazarus and Folkman (1984), who initiated most of the research into coping, distinguished between emotion-focused and problem-focused problem-solving.

Emotion-focused coping

This aims to alleviate distress by focusing on ways of reducing feelings of tension. It tends to be used when people feel the stressor can't be changed and must be endured. Techniques include relaxation methods that can be used to gain control of tension, help sleep, or control anxiety. It is possible to learn how to block out anxious thoughts, and to stop worrying about events that cannot be changed.

The process of sharing the stress by talking about events and feelings can also be helpful. The chance to talk about their worries, however, is not available for some people. Work may present no informal or formal opportunities to discuss tensions, and unless a supportive partner or relative is available to listen, there may be no chance to discuss such feelings.

Confronting is another emotion-focused method. It can be used positively or negatively. Getting angry and releasing a lot of emotion when confronting others may not be helpful; it will not solve the problem, and only leads to a discharge of feelings that goes nowhere. But if confrontation results in constructively sharing feelings it can be helpful. Loss of temper may make the situation worse, but calm determination and assertion can be constructive.

Methods of self-control can similarly be used positively or negatively. Self-control that reduces the level of anger or anxiety so the situation can be managed is helpful. But if unhappy feelings are contained and never allowed to surface they may eventually emerge as stress-related physical conditions and psychosomatic symptoms.

Problem-focused coping

This approach tries to solve the problems that are causing the stress by doing something to help reduce the stress and increase the sense of well-being. It is used when people feel something constructive can be done. Increasing motivation by setting small targets and then evaluating progress and congratulating oneself is very effective. Trying to find out more about the problem and obtain knowledge from colleagues, books, tutors, or management, can provide a sense of control and awareness. All of these efforts involve active problem-solving and a change in behaviour.

Some health professionals leave their jobs because of the stress at work, which is a perfectly reasonable way of solving the problem. What is important is that the person understands the reason for resigning, and does not feel it reflects inadequacy on their part. Giving feedback to the organization about the reasons for leaving, and identifying the unreasonable level of stress, and its causes may help the organization to look at ways to reduce the level of staff stress.

A number of other coping strategies exist. Behaviourally-based coping methods include palliatives like eating chocolates, smoking, drinking alcohol, or taking drugs or medication. These are all regularly used, but do not help with long-term or chronic stress. Such palliative measures can add to feelings of unhappiness because of the problems they bring with them – weight gain, drinking or smoking too much, or drug addiction. Taking exercise, planning social events, or starting a new hobby are all effective ways of increasing a personal sense of well-being away from work.

Carver *et al.*, (1989) have described 13 methods of coping. Any single response is adaptive for some people in some situations – there are no universally adaptive responses which are suitable for everyone all of the time.

➤ Active coping: problem-focused.

➤ Planning: thinking of strategies and steps to handle the problem.

➤ Suppression of competing activities: stopping other projects in order to handle the stress.

➤ Restraint coping: waiting for the right time to act.

➤ Seeking practical social support: getting advice and information.

➤ Seeking emotional social support: eliciting sympathy or under-standing.

➤ Focusing on and venting emotion.

➤ Behavioural disengagement: giving up.

➤ Mental disengagement: activities that distract from the stressor.

➤ Positive reinterpretation and growth: construing the stressful situation positively in order to actively problem-solve.

➤ Denial: refusal to believe in the stressor; acting as if it is not real.

➤ Acceptance: changes realistically made to accommodate the stressor.

➤ Turning to religion.

Brown Ceslowitz (1989) studied the relationship between coping strategies and burn-out in 150 nurses by measuring emotional exhaustion, depersonalization, and personal accomplishment. The Ways of Coping Scale (Folkman *et al.*, 1986) is shown in Table 8.1.

Table 8.1 *Ways of Coping Scale (Folkman* et al., *1986)*

Confronting	Accepting responsibility
Distancing	Planful problem-solving
Self-controlling	Escape/avoidance
Seeking social support	Positive reappraisal

Nurses who reduce their feelings of tension by relaxation or positive reappraisal of the situation, who ask for social support, and are able to use some self-controlling strategies are less likely to suffer from burn-out. Nurses who try to avoid the stress by wishful thinking, denial of the problems, the use of palliative measures, and self-controlling strategies that restrict their use of social support, and who confront problems are more likely to burn-out. Some methods, like planning problem-solving, seeking social support, and positive reappraisal, tend to elicit more social support than confronting and predominantly self-controlling methods do. The type of coping strategy used may therefore facilitate more positive feedback, which in turn helps alleviate the feelings of stress.

   Problem-solving may be related to the primary appraisal process. Nurses with lower burn-out scores may perceive stressful situations as more amenable to change, or may perceive their coping resources as adequate. But if the appraisal results in the nurse feeling unable to change the situation or feeling inadequate, they are more likely to use escape–avoidance methods of coping, a method used more by those nurses who experience burn-out (Folkman *et al.*, 1986).

Activity

Below are listed different coping methods (vertical scale) and different types of coping (horizontal scale). Tick the appropriate headings for each, and identify which ones you use at work and at home. Add any more you can think of.

Coping Methods	Types of coping		
	Emotional	**Behavioural**	**Problem-solving**
Smoking	—	—	—
Relaxation techniques	—	—	—
Going out with friends	—	—	—
Avoiding the problem or person	—	—	—
Information seeking	—	—	—
Giving yourself a treat	—	—	—
Taking exercise	—	—	—
Crying	—	—	—
Talking with a senior	—	—	—
Complaining to colleagues/friends	—	—	—
Keeping worries to yourself	—	—	—
Anticipating problems	—	—	—
Praying	—	—	—
Looking on the bright side	—	—	—
Leaving the job	—	—	—
Congratulating yourself	—	—	—
Setting small goals	—	—	—
Ignoring stress	—	—	—

Effective coping

Effective coping requires a clear analysis of the type of stress being experienced, and how it originates. Often stress arises from complex problems, and simple answers are not suitable. First, assessing whether the stress is part of an internal response or whether it is arising from external pressure is important. Secondly, it is necessary to believe change is possible in order to plan stress-coping strategies. The strategy to combat stress may take in several aspects:

Strengthening internal resources

This can include relaxation training, increasing physical exercise, modifying diet, assessing reliance on medication, improving assertiveness, improving communication skills, planning time management, and career planning.

Assessing stress at work

Team-building activities may need to be introduced to develop a support system. Team support group meetings can provide space and time for staff to release their fears and anxieties at work. Such meetings demonstrate to staff that their emotional needs are important and recognized.

The organization of the meetings can vary according to the needs of the team; they may be irregular – when needed – or regular events. All ward staff may meet together, or, initially, separate meetings for junior and senior staff can be arranged in order to allow junior staff to express themselves freely. Topics for discussion can vary from upset that someone is leaving, problems in communication, worries over particular patients or attitudes of medical colleagues, to concerns about staffing levels and work load. A suggestion box might be used so that the agenda is not always set by the senior nurse or the doctor.

It may be difficult to find the time in a busy schedule to devote to such meetings, but if morale on a team is low, or if there is high staff turnover and a lot of absenteeism, then stress is high and solutions are required. If such support groups are seen as being imposed from outside, or if team members do not feel safe to represent their true views, then they can fail.

Assessment of the management structure

This may identify areas of poor support, lack of a sense of direction, or a general feeling that there is a poor level of confidence. Talking with the ward sister or nurse manager may start to identify areas where stress can be relieved. A lack of cohesion can develop when there is a poor sense of leadership in a team. Similarly, team members can feel isolated and worried about a lack of good and close supervision, particularly if they are working in ways, or with problems and patients, of which they have little experience.

The organizational structure

This may be out of synchronization with the changing needs and roles of nurses. Work at a structural level may be required in terms of pay and conditions, shift-work patterns, hours, levels of accepted responsibility, and working practices. Change at this level is very slow and cumbersome, and may take many years.

Stress inoculation

Stress inoculation is a way of providing information about stressful experiences and events before they happen. It involves learning how to cope with patient-based stress more effectively, and increasing tolerance to these difficult experiences. Health professionals who are able to anticipate areas of stress are often better at managing the stress when it occurs. In daily clinical work there are a number of topics that can be identified as potentially stressful. For example, talking with dying children should be considered before it is faced in daily work. Deformities and disabilities, child abuse and sexual abuse, and the handling of difficult children are all issues that should be raised in advance.

Hurtig and Stewin (1990) carried out an experimental study to investigate the effects of a death-education programme and personal experiences of death on the attitudes of nursing students. The death-education programme aimed to increase the students' awareness of their feelings about their own death, as well as death in general. Lectures, films, and group discussions were used to present topics about death. This approach was compared to an experiential group, where a personal focus involved death-awareness exercises, music, drawing, and encounters between students. Students who had not experienced death personally found the experiential group more effective than the other approach, but students who had experienced death found it had a negative effect. This indicates the importance in

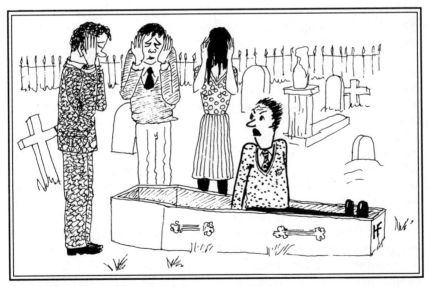

I think this is carrying the 'Death Education' programme a bit far.

assessing the individual needs of students. Inexperienced students may benefit from an experiential method in order to help them to encounter the thought of death, while death experienced students may require a cognitive approach initially so that they can confront their death concerns in a more indirect way. Students who have unresolved thoughts and feelings about a past death experience may require individual help.

Self-assertiveness

We all experience situations where we have different opinions to, or disagreements with, colleagues, which can create feelings of distress or resentment. How we manage such situations affects how we feel about ourselves, and how others feel about us.

Some people react to conflicts by not saying anything and avoiding the problem, which often leaves them feeling unhappy or angry, and can contribute to a lowering of self esteem. This is a passive way of reacting. Other people may launch into an attack by being critical and blaming in their response. Sometimes this is mistaken for assertive behaviour, but it is really aggressive behaviour. The aim is to belittle and blame the other person. It is outwardly expressive, but avoids taking responsibility for what is happening. Another method is to send a mixed message of anger couched in avoidance. For example, showing non-verbal anger by stamping around and being sulky, and then smiling sweetly at the person or saying nothing is the matter when asked. This is passive-avoidance behaviour, and may be used with people in authority because of a feeling of powerlessness. It is a way of withholding overt blame or criticism, but sends the message covertly.

Assertive behaviour enables direct communication with the other person, letting them know the effect of what they have said or done. It does not aim to blame or criticize, but to share the effect of their behaviour with them. One way of doing this is to use 'I' statements, for example, 'I feel hurt by what you just said', rather than 'you' messages, which put the blame on the other person for how we are feeling: 'You have hurt me by saying that'. Such statements make us think about what we are feeling. We learn to take responsibility for our feelings and to communicate them, rather than blame the other person for the way we feel. Changing ways of communicating takes effort and practice. Thinking about past events and rehearsing assertive ways of behaving helps build the skill of assertiveness. Practising with friends in a role-play can provide a way of testing out what to say. Sometimes it is easiest to start by making positive statements about how other people make you feel. To do this, you need to be able to recognize your feelings, label them, and then share them. To be able to tell other people what you admire or respect about them is one way of making them feel happy; it is also the first stage in being able to communicate your feelings to others.

Being assertive is not just about angry or resentful feelings, but includes the ability to give information to others about ourselves, seek information when we need it, and ask for others' opinions. Giving and receiving criticism in a constructive manner is also part of assertive behaviour, and may not be as painful or as embarrassing as it can be if criticism is destructive and undermining. To give constructive criticism we need to be able to point out others' good points, specifically describe the behaviour we feel should be changed, and help the person to think of solutions. What we say should be helpful, not hurtful.

Exercise

The next time someone upsets you, for example, when a fellow nurse asks you to serve lunches for the fourth time this week, think of a way of telling them how you feel and why you feel that way by using only 'I' statements, for example, 'I feel really fed up when I'm left to do most of the work. It makes me want to not work with you.'

It is very easy to fall into blaming the other person for how we feel: 'You make me really angry. You never do your fair share, and you always expect me to do it for you.' This aggressive statement blames the other person, which will either make them defensive or react aggressively. If you use the first statement, you will have a better chance of being heard. If your colleague wants to please you and keep on friendly terms then they will change their behaviour; if they choose not to change, then you may need to consider other solutions like splitting the work load to define areas of responsibility.

Summary

Nurses need to be aware of the effects of the stresses that are an integral part of the nursing role. These stresses can be interpersonal difficulties at work, organizational, patient or environmental stress, and can be compounded by stress in personal life.

Methods of coping with stress can be emotional, behavioural or problem focused. Some of these methods may not be effective so nurses need to consciously develop coping styles that can meet the pressures of work. Assessment of whether stress is due to internal or external pressure is important before coping strategies can be planned. These include strengthening internal resources, support stress reducing measures in the team, and examining the stress related to the management structure of the team.

The emotionally charged nature of nursing staff requires some stress inoculation training in order to prepare students for the realities of life. It is also necessary for all staff to learn how to be self-assertive and to be able to express their views clearly and constructively so that problems are expressed and managed openly and clearly.

Postscript: Ethical issues in nursing

Ethical and moral issues are common in nursing practice. They may be dramatic dilemmas, such as decisions to terminate treatment on ill children and babies, or they may involve daily decisions about which patient to visit in an overstretched community resource. There is a code of professional conduct for nurses which lists specific norms of behaviour that apply to the profession. These rules and guidelines provide the structure for daily practice but do not take the place of moral awareness (Van Hooft, 1990).

The development of caring

As a 'caring' profession, nursing is about being able to care for ill patients and alleviate suffering in the best possible way. This is the basis of a nurse's moral education. If a nurse feels uninterested in this basic nursing task, and is doing the job for the pay or because there was no other clear career option at the time, their values and attitudes may be in conflict with the professional attitude that is necessary to face complex moral and ethical decisions. The nurse has a task to uphold basic human values in a situation where patients are vulnerable and dependent. A humanitarian attitude is required, especially when technology and efficiency may have priority. The growth of nurses' moral and ethical awareness is based on the development of caring attitudes. This involves understanding the needs of the children and families in their care through humanitarianism and compassion which is based on empathy and respect for others' needs when they are most vulnerable and defenceless.

Illness brings with it pain, disfigurement, helplessness, distorted reactions, and sometimes bizarre and unpleasant behaviour that is frightening and irrational. Nurses need to be as aware of health as of illness, realizing that for each patient this period of illness is not their only life experience. The child is a member of a family, society, and culture, which provides a largely unknown set of relationships and experiences outside their nursing contact. How the nurse behaves towards the child and their parents will affect them and be part of their life experience forever. A child's illness in a family's life can carry powerful and painful memories and experiences; the nurse's behaviour

215

can be extremely significant at such a vulnerable and sensitive period in the child's life.

Ethical concepts

The way in which nurses demonstrate their value of patients' rights, freedom, and equality reflects their view of human dignity. This links with ideas discussed in Chapter 2 regarding the provision of equal nursing care across different sectors of the community. It is also relevant to Chapter 6 regarding helping children to undergo painful procedures, and gaining their consent to treatment, as well as Chapter 7, in which the needs of the dying child and their family are discussed. This basic view of human dignity underlies the whole reason for this book: to help the nurse to identify the differences in people's needs, their individuality, and their special qualities, in order to use insight and awareness.

The nurse's commitment to caring for the health and welfare of patients needs to be well founded. It also must be well defended against the desensitizing influences of institutional routines and pressures, and high work load. It is only too easy for emotional and stress reactions to interfere with the nurse's ability to care for patients. Nurses may be unaware of how their sensitivity has become dulled to the agony that the parents of a sick child are experiencing – because they have faced the same situation hundreds of times. It is easy to feel irritated when a child will not co-operate in the necessary nursing treatment when there is a long list of jobs to complete. It is easy to retreat back into the demands of routine rather than to adapt circumstances to the particular needs of patients; it is safer to protect ourselves from the pain of making – and losing – a close relationship with a sick or dying child with the excuse that there is too much to do. It is by balancing job pressures with moral awareness that nurses are able to behave in ways that enhance the dignity of sick children and their families.

Trust

We are taught from childhood that telling the truth is correct. But how often do people in positions of power, who think they know best, avoid telling the truth? What happens when telling the truth to a patient comes into conflict with the basic caring principles?

In the health care professions the issues of truth telling and providing the best form of treatment are interwoven, and can create a moral dilemma. Is it ever in the best interests of patients *not* to know the truth about their illness? Should children *always be* told their diagnosis and prognosis? Should parents have the right to veto nurses telling the truth to a child who is asking for information? Perhaps it is not possible to generalize about such conflicts; perhaps 'yes' or 'no' responses are not enough.

Freedom

Our society greatly values the freedom and autonomy of the individual to behave as he or she chooses within the law. But ill patients are not free; they are constrained by their illness and are dependent on others for care and protection. The freedom and autonomy of each patient is a difficult issue on a busy and overcrowded ward, where it is easier for the nurses if the patients fit into the institutional regime. While nursing has gradually loosened the rigid structure of the daily ward routine to the benefit ot the individual needs of patients, there are still conflicts. What happens if a child wants to go to the hospital play centre but needs a nurse to monitor them and there is no spare nurse on the ward? Should a parent be allowed to take their child out of the ward for a walk around the local park? Should a parent be allowed to give their child the necessary medication while in hospital, or should nurses insist on doing it because 'that is the rule'?

The constraints placed on children while in hospital have lessened dramatically in recent nursing history. Children are no longer expected to stay in or on their beds if they can get up; portable lines are used to provide as much physical freedom as possible; play areas are provided to keep children amused and occupied. Although nurses today may feel they have the best interests and the safety of the children at heart, nurses at the turn of the century also felt this, and consider the changes since then.

Where possible, nursing is adopting a patient-based rather than a task-centred approach. This is a psychological and humanitarian approach that recognizes the individual emotional needs of the patients. It aims to reduce the number of nurses that each patient comes into contact with, and to allow closer relationships to develop between patient and nurse.

In the past, task-centred nursing identified the daily tasks on the ward and allocated these across the team, regardless of the individual needs of the patients. Interestingly, the arguments for and against a change in nursing practice highlight the difference in attitude between awareness of the emotional needs of the patient and nurse versus the number of tasks to be completed. How efficient and how cost effective is this change in approach? How would you evaluate the possibility of improved care for the patient?

The rights of the individual

Health care professionals face many situations where they exert control over the right to life of their patients. Issues surrounding abortion, euthanasia, and terminating active treatment are the classic major ethical issues. Different religions and different sectors of the community have strong views about this.

Paediatric nurses may be faced with the issue of involvement in terminating active treatment of a severely disabled baby or ill child (Kuhse and Singer, 1985). Should children always be saved, regardless of their quality of life? Can we equate the fact that a child's life is preserved with the fact that they may then live in continual pain, with severe physical or mental disabilities, and with severe restrictions on the possibility of ever living a normal life? Should children be made to undergo repeated and severely painful and unpleasant medical procedures with little evidence of their effectiveness, or low positive outcome rates? How can a baby be refused admission to a hospital on financial grounds, knowing that the baby will probably be severely disabled by any delay, or even die?

There are no simple answers to any of these questions. All we can do is to be aware of the dilemmas and conflicts involved, discuss them, and try to make decisions that best meet humanitarian considerations.

Moral awareness

Moral awareness should lead to a sense of personal confidence, insight, and sensitivity that enables responsible decisions to be made. To act decisively in a morally difficult or ambiguous situation fulfils our sense of moral commitment. We may need to overcome our fears, shyness, social or cultural prejudice, peer pressure, or professional pressure in order to act in a way we feel is ethical. The strength to act in accordance with our personal views is always an ethical action (Van Hooft, 1990).

Learning ethical behaviour is not about learning the rules or avoiding being legally liable for misconduct. It is learning how to act in difficult and stressful situations where there are no clear guidelines. We learn how to behave by watching others. Demonstration and modelling of sensitivity and caring from fellow nurses and seniors during their daily routine is one way of absorbing the nursing ethos. The managing of heavy caseloads and difficult patients or families in a sensitive and caring manner can be taught more by example than by learning guidelines or principles. Once this approach is applied to everyday work it becomes a habit that is repeated. It is then possible to reflect on behaviour and to apply moral behaviour to more complex and difficult situations.

It is extremely difficult to consider ethical and moral behaviour in isolation and without a basic attitudinal position that has been developed in the practical situation. The strength of will and conviction to act well comes from the knowledge that we acted well in the past, and that we are behaving in a way that fits with our personal attitudes and motivations.

The confidence about how to behave and react in ordinary or unusual situations develops over time and with experience. Watching others, practising, reflecting on what has happened, and self-understanding form the basis of a moral stance. This does not mean we necessarily know how to behave in all situations, but it is possible to act in accordance with our underlying caring attitudes so we can feel content and live with our actions and decisions. This allows a flexible and thoughtful approach to complex decisions, rather that a strict adherence to an underdeveloped code of behaviour that is poorly understood and may be misapplied. No single code or rule applies to all situations. We have to take responsibility within ourselves for our actions because we have to live with ourselves. It is not possible to hide behind rules that another creates, and we cannot pass the ethical responsibility on to anyone else. We may not act the same way each time, but we should be able to do what we think is best according to the circumstances.

Moral awareness and the future

The way in which problems are solved will either enhance or undermine personal confidence. In order to be aware of problems in the daily structure and routine it is necessary to enhance our sensitivity and be prepared to help to improve nursing care for the benefit of patients. Being constructively critical of the daily routine indicates an openness to suggestions for change and improvement. The responsibility of a caring nurse is always to try to improve the standards of nursing care for the benefit of patients. By considering your patients' rights and by trying to fulfil them in the best possible way, you may trigger off a new style of nursing practice or management that beneficially affects the whole of the nursing profession and its patients.

Sumary

Inevitably, ethical issues arise in nursing. Nurses who are highly stressed are unlikely to be able to demonstrate compassion and empathy for their patients. The ethical concepts of truth, freedom, and personal rights are inextricably bound up with the health professional's ability to view each patient as an individual, with a complex psychological history, and a unique future. The nurse plays a significant role in interpreting the changing values and attitudes in society, and applying the growing knowledge about psychological needs in their daily work. To do this successfully, all health professionals need frequently to examine and evaluate their own behaviour, attitudes and expectations.

References

Achenbach, T. M. & Edelbrock, C. S. (1983) *The Child Behaviour Checklist Manual*. Burlington, VT, The University of Vermont.

Adams, D. W. & Deveau, E. J. (1986) Helping dying adolescents: needs and responses. In C. A. Corr and J. N. McNeil (eds) (1986) *Adolescence and Death*. New York, Springer Publishing Company.

Ainsworth, M. D. S., Blehar, M. C., Waters, E. & Wall, S. (1978) *Patterns of Attachment: a Psychological Study of the Strange Situation*. Hillsdale, NJ, Lawrence Erlbaum.

Allen, L. & Zigler, E. (1986) Psychological adjustment of seriously ill children. *Journal of the American Academy of Child and Adolescent Psychiatry, 25*, 708–712.

Anderson, J. (1986) Ethnicity and illness experiences: ideological structures and the health care delivery system. *Social Science and Medicine, 22*, 1277–1283.

Ashton, J. & Seymour, H. (1988) *The New Public Health*. Milton Keynes, Open University Press.

Azar, S. T., Barnes, K. T. & Twentyman, C. T. (1988) Developmental outcomes in abused children; consequences of parental abuse or a more general breakdown in caregiver behaviour? *Behaviour Therapist, 11*, 27–32.

Bailey, R. D. (1985) *Coping with Stress in Caring*. Oxford, Blackwell Scientific Publications.

Baker, T. & Duncan, S. (1985) Child sexual abuse – a study of prevalence in Great Britain. *Journal of Child Abuse and Neglect, 9*, 457–567.

Barker, P. (1988) *Basic Child Psychiatry*, 5th ed. Oxford, Blackwell Scientific Publications.

Baron-Cohen, S. (1989) The autistic child's theory of mind: a case of specific developmental delay. *Journal of Child Psychology and Psychiatry, 30*, 285–297.

Baron-Cohen, S., Leslie, A. M. & Frith, U. (1986) Mechanical, behavioural and intentional understanding of picture stories in autistic children. *British Journal of Developmental Psychology, 4*, 113–125.

Baumrind, D. (1980) New directions in socialization research. *American Psychologist, 35*, 639–657.

Beale, J. A. (1989) The effects of demonstration of the Brazelton Neonatal Assessment Scale on paternal–infant relationship. *Issues in Perinatology, 16*, 18–22.

Beale, J. A. (1991) Methodological issues in conducting research on parent–infant attachment. *Journal of Pediatric Nursing, 6*, 11–15.

Beezley-Mrazek, P. & Kempe, C. H. (1981) *Sexually Abused Children on their Families*. Oxford, Pergamon Press.

Behar, L. & Stringfield, S. (1974) A behaviour rating scale for the pre-school child. *Developmental Psychology, 10*, 601–610.

Bellman, M. (1966) Studies on encopresis. *Acta Paediatrica Scandinavica*, Supplement 170.

Belsky, J. (1985) Experimenting with the family in the newborn period. *Child Development, 56*, 407–414.

Bentovim, A., Elton, A., Hildebrand, J., Tranter, M. & Vizard, E. (1988) *Child Sexual Abuse within the Family: Assessment and Treatment*. London, Wright.

Berden, G. F. M. G., Althaus, M. & Verhulst, F. C. (1990) Major life events and changes in the behavioural functioning of children. *Journal of Child Psychology and Psychiatry, 31*, 949–961.

Berreuta-Clement, J. R., Schweinhart, L. J., Barnett, W. S., Epstein, A. S. & Weikart, D. P. (1984) *Changed lives: the effects of the Perry preschoool programs on youths through age 19.* Yipsilanti, Michigan, The High/Scope Press.

Beyer, J. E. & Aradine, C. R. (1986) Convergent and discriminant validity of a self report measure of pain intensity for children. *Children's Health Care, 16,* 274–282.

Billingham, K. (1989) 45 Cope Street: Working in partnership with parents. *Health Visitor, 62,* 156–157.

Blacher, J. (1984) Sequential stages of parental adjustment to the birth of a child with handicaps: fact or artefact. *Mental Retardation, 22,* 55–69.

Black, D. & Urbanowitz, M. (1987) Family intervention with bereaved children. *Journal of Child Psychology and Psychiatry, 28,* 467–476.

Blagg, N. R. & Yule, W. (1984) The behavioural treatment of school refusal: a comparative study. *Behaviour Research and Therapy, 22,* 119–127.

Block, J., Block, J. H. & Gjerde, P. (1988) Parental functioning and home environment in families of divorce: prospective and concurrent analyses. *Journal of the American Academy of Child and Adolescent Psychiatry, 27,* 207–213.

Bolig, R. (1984) Play in hospital settings. In T. D. Yawkey & A. D. Pellegrini (eds) *Child's Play: Developmental and Applied.* Hillsdale, NJ, Lawrence Erlbaum.

Bowlby, J. (1953) *Child Care and the Growth of Love.* Harmondsworth, Penguin.

Bowlby, J. (1969) *Attachment and Loss, Vol. 1: Attachment.* London, Hogarth Press.

Bowlby, J. (1973) *Attachment and Loss, Vol. 2: Separation, Anxiety and Anger.* New York, Basic Books.

Bowling, A. & Stilwell, B. (1988) *The Nurse in Family Practice.* London, Scutari Press.

Brain, D. J. & Maclay, I. (1968) Controlled study of mothers and children in hospital. *British Medical Journal, 1,* 278–280.

Breslau, N., Weitzman, M. & Messenger, K. (1981) Psychological functioning of siblings of disabled children. *Pediatrics, 67,* 344–353.

Brett, K. M. (1988) Sibling response to chronic childhood disorders: research perspectives and practice implications. *Issues in Comprehensive Pediatric Nursing, 11,* 43–57.

Brewster, A. B. (1982) Chronically ill hospitalized children's concepts of their illness. *Pediatrics, 69,* 355–362.

Brinker, R. P. & Lewis, M. (1982) Discovering the competent handicapped infant: a process approach to assessment and intervention. *Topics in Early Childhood Special Education, 2,* 1–16.

Browne, K., Davies, C. & Stratton, P. (eds) (1988) *Early Prediction and Prevention of Child Abuse.* Chichester, Wiley.

Browne, K. & Saqi, S. (1987) Parent–child interaction in child abusing families: possible causes and consequences. In P. Mahe (ed.) *Child Abuse: An Educational Perspective.* Oxford, Blackwell.

Browne, K. Saqi, S. (1988a) Approaches to screening for child abuse and neglect. In K. Browne, C. Davies & P. Stratton (eds) (1988) *Early Prediction and Prevention of Child Abuse.* Chichester, Wiley.

Browne, K. & Saqi, S. (1988b) Mother infant interaction and attachment in physically abusing families. *Journal of Reproductive and Infant Psychology, 6.*

Browne, K. D. & Stevenson, J. (1983) A checklist for completion by health visitors to identify children 'at risk' for child abuse. Report to Surrey County Area Review Committee on Child Abuse (unpubl.)

Cairns, C., Clark, M., Smith, S. & Lansky, S. (1979) Adaptation of siblings to childhood malignancy. *Journal of Pediatrics, 95,* 484–487.

Carey, S. (1985) *Conceptual Change in Childhood*. Cambridge, MA, MIT.

Carpenter, A. (1990) Sleep problems: a group approach. *Health Visitor*, *63*, 305–307.

Carr, J. (1988) Six weeks to twenty-one years old: a longitudinal study of children with Down's syndrome and their families. *Journal of Child Psychology and Psychiatry*, *29*, 407–433.

Carver, C. S., Scheier, M. F. & Weintraub, J. M. (1989) Assessing coping strategies: a theoretically based approach. *Journal of Personality and Social Psychology*, *56*, 267–83.

Central Statistical Office (1991) *Social Trends*, No. 21. London, HMSO.

Christ, G., Siegel, K., Mesagno, F. & Langosch, D. (1991) A preventive intervention program for bereaved children: problems of implementation. *American Journal of Orthopsychiatry*, *61*, 168–178.

Cleary, J., Gray, O. P., Hall, D. J., Rowlandson, P. H., Sainsbury, C. P. O. & Davies, M. M. (1986) Parental involvement in the lives of children in hospital. *Archives of Disease in Childhood*, *61*, 779–787.

Conger, J. J. & Peterson, A. C. (1984) *Adolescence and Youth*, 3rd ed. New York, Harper and Row.

Cooper, C. L. & Mitchell, S. (1990) Nurses under stress: a reliability and validity study of the NSI. *Stress Medicine*, *6*, 21–24.

Corr, C. & McNeil, J. (eds) (1986) *Adolescence and Death*. New York, Springer Publishing Company.

Cox, T. (1978) *Stress*. London, Macmillan.

Cox, A, Holbrook, D. & Rutter, M. (1981a) Psychiatric inteviewing techniques VI. Experimental study: eliciting feelings. *British Journal of Psychiatry*, *139*, 144–152.

Cox, A., Rutter, M. & Holbrook, D. (1981b) Psychiatric interviewing techniques V. Experimental study: eliciting factual information. *British Journal of Psychiatry*, *139*, 29–37.

Creighton, S. J. (1988) The incidence of child abuse and neglect. In K. Browne, C. Davies & P. Stratton (eds) *Early Prediction and Prevention of Child Abuse* Chichester, Wiley.

Cunningham, C. C., Aumonier, M. E. & Sloper, P. (1982a) Health visitor support for families with Down's syndrome infants. *Child: Care, Health and Development*, *8*, 1–19.

Cunningham, C. C., Aumonier, M. E. & Sloper, P. (1982b) Health visitor services for families with a Down's syndrome infant. *Child: Care, Health and Development*, *8*, 311–326.

Cunningham, C. C. & Davis, H. (1985) *Working with Parents: Frameworks for Collaboration*. Milton Keynes, Open University Press.

Czajkowski, D. R. & Koocher, G. P. (1987) Medical compliance and coping with cystic fibrosis *Journal of Child Psychology and Psychiatry*, *28*, 311–321.

Darlington, R. B., Royce, J. M., Snipper, A. S., Murray, H. W. & Lazar, I. (1980) Preschool programs and later school competence of children from low-income families. *Science*, *208*, 202–204.

Deatrick, J. A. & Knafl, K. A. (1990) Management behaviours: day-to-day adjustments to childhood chronic conditions. *Journal of Pediatric Nursing*, *5*, 15–22.

Deatrick, J. A., Knafl, K. A. & Walsh, M. (1988) The process of parenting a child with a disability. Normalization through accommodations. *The Journal of Advanced Nursing*, *13*, 15–21.

DeJonge, G. A. (1973) Epidemiology of enuresis: a survey of the literature. In I. Kolvin, R. C. MacKeith & S. R. Meadow (eds) *Bladder Control and Enuresis* (Clinics in Developmental Medicine nos 48/49). London, Heinemann.

Department of Health (1989) *The Children Act.* London, HMSO.

Department of Health (1991) *Welfare of Children and Young People in Hospital.* London, HMSO.

Department of Health and Social Security (DHSS) (1986) *Neighbourhood Nursing – Focus for Care* (The Cumberledge Report). London, HMSO.

Dische, S., Yule, W., Corebett, J. A. & Hand, D. (1983) Childhood nocturnal enuresis: factors associated with outcome of treatment with an enuresis alarm. *Developmental Medicine and Child Neurology, 25,* 67–80.

Dominica, F. (1987) The role of the hospice for the hospice for the dying child. *British Journal of Hospital Medicine, 38,* 334–342.

Donovan, C. F. (1984) Life changes – divorce. *British Medical Journal, 289,* 597–600.

Douglas, J. (1991) Psychologically based eating problems in young children. *Maternal and Child Health, 16,* 251–254.

Douglas, J. & Richman, N. (1984) *My Child Won't Sleep.* Harmondsworth, Penguin.

Douglas, S. (1985) The most stressful speciality? *Nursing Mirror, 161,* 32–34.

Egger, J., Carter, C. M., Graham, P. J., Gumley, D. & Southill,. J. F. (1985) Controlled trial of oligoantigenic treatment in the hyperkinetic syndrome. *Lancet,* (i) 540–545.

Eiser, C. (1990a) Psychological effects of chronic disease. *Journal of Child Psychology and Psychiatry, 31,* 85–98.

Eiser, C. (1990b) *Chronic Childhood Disease: an Introduction to Psychological Theory and Research.* Cambridge, Cambridge University Press.

Eiser, C. & Patterson, D. (1983) Slugs and snails and puppy dog tails – children's ideas about the inside of their bodies. *Child: Care, Health and Development, 9,* 233–240.

Elliott, C. H. & Olson, R. A. (1983) The management of children's behavioural distress in response to painful medical treatment for burn injuries. *Behaviour Research and Therapy, 21,* 675–683.

Fehrenbach, A. M. B. & Peterson, L. (1989) Parental problem solving skills, stress and dietary compliance in phenylketonuria. *Journal of Consulting and Clinical Psychology, 57,* 237–241.

Fletcher, B. (1981) Psychological upset in post-hospitalised children: a review of the literature. *Maternal Child Nursing Journal, 10,* 185–195.

Folkman, S., Lazarus, R. S., Gruen, R. J. & Delongis, A. (1986) Appraisal, coping, health status and psychological symptoms. *Journal of Personality and Social Psychology, 50,* 571–579.

Forehand, R. L. & McMahon, R. J. (1981) *Helping the Non-compliant Child: a Clinician's Guide.* New York, Guilford.

Forness, S. R. & Hecht, B. (1988) Special education for handicapped and disabled children: classification, progress and trends. *Journal of Pediatric Nursing, 3,* 75–85.

Forrest, G., Claridge, R. & Baum, J. (1981) Practical management of perinatal death. *British Medical Journal, 282,* 31–32.

Fraser, W. I. & Rao, J. M. (1991) Recent studies of mentally handicapped young people's behaviour. *J. Child Psychology and Psychiatry, 32,* 79–109.

Friedrich, W. N., Wilturner, L. T. & Cohen, D. S. (1985) Coping resources and parenting mentally retarded children. *American Journal of Mental Deficiency, 90,* 130–139.

Gaffney, A. & Dunn, E. A. (1986) Developmental aspects of children's definitions of pain. *Pain 26,* 105–117.

Gallo, A. M. (1990) Family management style in juvenile diabetes: a case illustration. *Journal of Pediatric Nursing, 5,* 23–32.

Garralda, M. E. Jameson, R. A., Reynolds, J. M. & Postlethwaite, J. R. (1988) Psychiatric adjustment in children with chronic renal failure. *Journal of Child Psychology and Psychiatry, 29,* 79–90.

Gath, A. M. (1972) The mental health of siblings of congenitally abnormal children. *Journal of Child Psychology and Psychiatry, 13,* 211–218.

Gibson, C. (1988) Perspectives in parental coping with a chronically ill child: the case of cystic fibrosis. *Issues in Comprehensive Nursing, 11,* 33–41.

Gillberg, C. (1990) Autism and pervasive developmental disorder. *Journal of Child Psychology and Psychiatry, 31,* 99–121.

Gillberg, C. (1991) Outcome in autism and autistic-like conditions. *Journal of the American Academy of Child and Adolescent Psychiatry, 30,* 375–381.

Goldberg, D. (1988) *General Health Questionnaire.* Windsor, N.F.E.R./Nelson.

Goodwin, S. (1987) Stress in health visiting. *Recent Advances in Nursing, 15,* 99–111.

Goodyer, I. M. (1990) Family relationships life events and childhood psychopathology. *Journal of Child Psychology and Psychiatry, 31,* 161–192.

Graziano, A. M., DeGiovanni, I. S. & Garcia, K. A. (1979) Behavioural treatment of children's fears: review. *Psychological Bulletin, 86,* 804–830.

Halliday, S., Meadow, S. R. & Berg, I. (1987) Successful management of daytime enuresis using alarm procedures: a randomly controlled trial. *Archives of Disease in Childhood, 62,* 132–137.

Hanks, H., Hobbs, C. & Wynne, J. (1988) Early signs and recognition of sexual abuse in the pre-school child In K. Browne, C. Davies & P. Stratton (eds) *Early Prediction and Prevention of Child Abuse.* Chichester, Wiley.

Harlow, H. F. (1959) The development of learning in rhesus monkeys. *American Scientist, 47,* 459–479.

Haslum, M. (1988) Length of preschool hospitalisation, multiple admissions and later educational attainment and behaviour. *Child: Care, Health and Development, 14,* 275–291.

Henderson, G. & Primeaux, M. (1981) *Transcultural Health Care.* London, Addison-Wesley.

Herbert, M. (1987) *Behavioural Treatment of Problem Children,* 2nd ed. London Academic Press.

Hersov, L. (1985) Faecal soiling. In M. Rutter & L. Hersov (eds) *Child and Adolescent Psychiatry: Modern Approaches,* Oxford Blackwell Scientific Publications.

Hetherington, E. M. (1989) Coping with family transitions: winners losers and survivors. *Child Development, 60,* 1–14.

Hewett, K. (1990) Assessment by health visitors of behavioural problems in pre-school children. In J. Stevenson (ed) *Health Visitor Based Services for Pre-school Children with Behaviour Problems.* Occasional Paper No. 2. Association of Child Psychology and Psychiatry.

Hipwell, A. E., Tyler P. A. & Wilson, C. M. (1989) Sources of stress and dissatisfaction among nurses in four hospital environments. *British Journal of Medical Psychology, 62,* 71–79.

Hiskins, G. (1981) How mothers help themselves. *Health Visitor, 54,* 108–111.

Hobson, R. P. (1988) Beyond cognition: a theory of autism. In G. Dawson (ed.) *Autism: New Perspectives on Diagnosis, Nature and Treatment.* New York, Guilford.

Hornsby, B. (1984) *Overcoming Dyslexia: a Straightforward Guide for Families and Teachers.* London, Martin Dunitz.

Howlin, P. & Rutter, M. (1987) *Treatment of Autistic Children.* New York, Wiley.

Hurtig, W. A. & Stewin, L. (1990) The effect of health education and experience on nursing students's attitudes towards death. *Journal of Advanced Nursing, 15*, 29–34.

Hyland, M. E. & Donaldson, M. L. (1989) *Psychological Care in Nursing Practice.* Harrow, Scutari Press.

Jay, S. M., Elliott, C. H., Ozalins, M., Olson, R. A. & Pruitt, S. D. (1985) Behavioural management of children's distress during painful medical procedures. *Behaviour Research and Therapy, 23*, 513–520.

Johnston, J. R., Kline, M. & Tscann, J. M. (1989) Ongoing post divorce conflict. *American Journal of Orthopsychiatry, 59*, 576–592.

Kane, B. (1979) Children's concept of death. *Journal of Genetic Psychology, 134*, 141–153.

Kashani, J. H., Ray, J. S. & Carlson, G. A. (1984) Depression and depression like states in pre-school age children in a child development unit. *American Journal of Psychiatry, 141*, 1397–1402.

Kaufman, J. & Zigler, E. (1987) Do abused children become abusive parents? *American Journal of Orthopsychiatry, 57*, 186–192.

Keane, A., Ducette, J. & Adler, D. C. (1985) Stress in ICU and non-ICU nurses. *Nursing Research, 34*, 231–236.

Kendall, P. C. & Braswell, L. (1985) *Cognitive-Behavioural Therapy for Impulsive Children.* New York, Guilford.

Kister, M. C. & Patterson, C. J. (1980) Children's conceptions of the causes of illness: understanding of contagion and use of immanent justice. *Child Development, 51*, 839–846.

Klaus, M. H. & Kennell, J. H. (1976) *Maternal–Infant Bonding.* St Louis, Mosby.

Knafl, K. A. & Deatrick, J. A. (1990) Family management style: concept analysis and development. *Journal of Pediatric Nursing, 5*, 4–14.

Kübler-Ross, E. (1983) *On Children and Death.* London, Souvenir Press.

Kuhse, H. & Singer, P. (1985) *Should the Baby Live? The Problem of Handicapped Infants.* Oxford, Oxford University Press.

Kuykendall, J. (1989) Death of a child – the worst kept secret around. In L. Sherr (ed.) *Death, Dying and Bereavement.* Oxford, Blackwell.

LaMontagne, L. L. (1987) Children's pre-operative coping: replication and extension. *Nursing Research, 36*, 163–167.

Landsdown, R. (1989) The care of the child facing death. *Process in Pediatric Surgery, 22*, 64–68.

Lansdown, R. & Benjamin, G. (1985) The development of the concept of death in children aged five to nine years. *Child: Care, Health and Development, 11*, 13–20.

Lattanzi, M. E. (1985) An approach to caring in caregiver concerns. In C. A. Corr & M. C. Corr (eds) *Hospice Approaches to Pediatric Care.* New York, Springer Publishing Company.

Lauer, M. E. & Camitta, B. M. (1980) Home care for dying children: a nursing model. *Journal of Pediatrics, 97*, 1032–1035.

Lavigne, J. V. & Ryan, M. (1979) Psychologic adjustment of siblings of children with chronic illness. *Pediatrics, 63*, 616–627.

Lazarus, R. S. & Folkman, S. (1984) *Stress, Appraisal and Coping.* New York, Springer Publishing Company.

Lerner, M. J., Haley, J. V., Hall, D. S. & McVarish, D. (1972) Hospital care by parent: an evaluative look. *Medical Care, 10*, 430–436.

Lewis, C. (1986) The role of the father in the human family. In W. Sluckin & M. Herbert (eds) *Parental Behaviour.* Oxford, Blackwell.

Manion, J. (1990) Preparing children for hospitalisation, procedures of surgery. In M. J. Craft & J. A. Denehy (eds) *Nursing Interventions for Infants and Children*. Philadelphia, W. B. Saunders.

Mawson, D., Marks, I., Ramm, L. & Stern, R. (1981) Guided mourning for morbid grief: a controlled study. *British Journal of Psychiatry, 138*, 185–193.

May, K. (1989) A new venture in health care. *Health Visitor, 62*, 211–213.

McCown, D. E. (1988) When children face death in a family. *Journal of Pediatric Health Care, 2*, 14–19.

McFarlane, A. C. (1988) Recent life events and psychiatric disorder in children: the interaction with preceding extreme adversity. *Journal of Child Psychology and Psychiatry, 29*, 677–691.

McFarlane, K. & Waterman, J. (1986) *Sexual Abuse of Young Children*. London, Holt, Rinehart & Winston.

Melamed, B. G., Dearborn, M. & Hermecz, D. A. (1983) Necessary considerations for surgery preparation: age and previous experience. *Psychosomatic Medicine, 45*, 517–525.

Mills, M., Puckering, C., Pound, A. & Cox, A. (1985) What is it about depressed mothers that influences their children's functioning? In J. Stevenson (ed.) *Recent Advances in Developmental Psychopathology*. Oxford, Pergamon.

Minuchin, S., Rosman, B. L. & Baker, E. R. L. (1978) *Psychosomatic Families*. Cambridge, MA, Harvard University Press.

Moulds, V., Hennessy, D. & Crack, P. (1983a) Innovations by a primary health care team: 1. Well-baby clinics by appointment. *Health Visitor, 56*, 295–296.

Moulds, V. Hennessy, D. & Crack, P. (1983b) Innovations by a primary health care team: 2. A post-natal group for first-time mothers. *Health Visitor, 56*, 296–297.

Moyer, A. (1989) Caring for a child with diabetes: the effect of specialist nurse care on parents' needs and concerns. *Journal of Advanced Nursing, 14*, 536–545.

Mulholland, C. (1987) *I'll Dance with the Rainbows*. Glasgow, Patrick.

Newson, J. & Newson, E. (1979) *Toys and Play Things*. Harmondsworth, Penguin.

Nichols, K. A., Springford, V. & Searl, J. (1981) An investigation of distress and discontent in various types of nursing. *Journal of Advanced Nursing, 6*, 311–338.

Nicol, A. R., Stretch, D. D., Fundudis, T., Smith, I. & Davison, I. (1987) The nature of mother and toddler problems – I. Development of a multiple criterion screen. *Journal of Child Psychology and Psychiatry, 28*, 739–754.

Offord, D. R. (1987) Prevention of behavioural and emotional disorders in children. *Journal of Child Psychology and Psychiatry, 28*, 9–21.

Offord, D. R., Boyle, M. H., Szatmari, P., Rae-Grant, N. I., Links, P. S., Cadman, D. T., Ryles, J. A., Crawford, J. W., Blum, H. M., Byrne, C., Thomas, H. & Woodward, C. A. (1987) Ontario Child Health Study – II. Six month prevalence of disorder and rates of service utilization. *Archives of General Psychiatry, 44*, 832–836.

Olness, K. (1989) Hypnotherapy: a cyberphysiologic strategy in pain management. *Pediatric Clinics of North America, 36*, 873–884.

Olness, K. N. & Gardner, G. C. (1988) *Hypnosis and Hypnotherapy with Children*. New York, Grune & Stratton.

Orr, J. (1985) The community dimension. In K. Luker & J. Orr (eds) *Health Visiting*. Oxford, Blackwell Scientific Publications.

Pagel, I. S. & Wittmann, M. E. (1986) Relationship of burnout to personal and job-related variables in acute-care pediatric setting. *Issues in Comprehensive Nursing, 9,* 131–143.

Patterson, G. R. (1982) *Coercive Family Process.* Oregon, Castalia, Eugene.

Perrin, E. C. & Gerrity, P. S. (1981) There's a demon in your belly: children's understanding of illness. *Pediatrics, 67,* 841–849.

Perrin, J. M. & MacLean, W. E. (1988) Children with chronic illness: the prevention of dysfunction. *Pediatric Clinics of North America, 35,* 1325–1337.

Peterson, L. (1989) Coping by children undergoing stressful medical procedures: some conceptual, methodological and therapeutic issues. *Journal of Consulting and Clinical Psychology, 57,* 380–387.

Pound, A. & Mills, M. (1985) A pilot evaluation of NEWPIN: a home visiting and befriending scheme in South London. *Newsletter of the Association for Child Psychology and Psychiatry, 7,* 13–15.

Powers, S., Dill, D., Houser, S., Noam, G. & Jacobsen, A. (1984) Coping strategies of families of seriously ill adolescents. *Journal of Early Adolescence, 5,* 101–113.

Puckering, C. (1989) Maternal Depression. *Journal of Child Psychology and Psychiatry, 30,* 807–817.

Quinton, D. & Rutter, M. (1976) Early hospital admissions and later disturbances of behaviour: an attempted replication of Douglas's findings. *Developmental Medicine and Child Neurology, 18,* 447–459.

Reichman, J. & Healey, W. (1983) Hearing disabilities and conductive hearing loss involving otitis media. *Journal of Hearing Disabilities, 16,* 272–278.

Reilly, T. P., Hasazi, J. E. & Bobd, L. A. (1983) Children's conceptions of death and personal mortality. *Journal of Pediatric Psychology, 8,* 21–31.

Richards, M. P. M. (1988) Parental divorce and children. In G. Burrows (ed.) *Handbook of Studies in Child Psychiatry.* Amsterdam, Elsevier.

Richman, N. (1977) Is a behaviour checklist for pre-school children useful? In P. J. Graham (ed.) *Epidemiological Approaches in Child Psychiatry.* London, Academic Press.

Richman, N. (1988) Feeding problems. In J. Douglas (ed) (1988) *Emotional and Behavioural Problems in Young Children. A multidisciplinary approach to identification management.* Windsor, NFER-Nelson.

Richman, N & Graham, P. (1971) A behavioural screening questionnaire for use with three-year-old children: preliminary findings. *Journal of Child Psychology and Psychiatry, 12,* 5–33.

Richman, N., Stevenson, J. & Graham, P. (1982) *Pre-school to School: a Behavioural Study.* London, Academic Press.

Richman, N., Douglas, J., Hunt, H., Lansdown, R. & Levere, R. (1985) Behavioural methods in the treatment of sleep disorders – a pilot study. *Journal of Child Psychology and Psychiatry, 26,* 581–591.

Ritchie, K. (1981) Research note: interactions in the families of epileptic children. *Journal of Child Psychology and Psychiatry, 22,* 65–71.

Roberts, J. (1988) Why are some families more vulnerable to child abuse? In K. Browne, C. Davies & P. Stratton (eds) *Early Prediction and Prevention of Child Abuse.* Chichester, Wiley.

Robins, L. N. (1991) Conduct disorder. *Journal of Child Psychology and Psychiatry, 32,* 193–213.

Rogers, C. R. (1951) *Client Centred Therapy.* Boston, MA, Houghton Mifflin.

Rosen, H. (1986) *Unspoken Grief: Coping with Childhood Sibling Loss.* Lexington, MA, Lexington Books.

Ross, D. M. & Ross, S. A. (1984) Childhood pain: the school aged child's viewpoint. *Pain, 20,* 179–191.

Rutter, M. (1981) *Maternal Deprivation Re-assessed*, 2nd ed. Harmondsworth, Penguin.

Rutter, M. (1981) Stress, coping in development: some issues and some questions. *Journal of Child Psychology and Psychiatry, 22,* 323–356.

Rutter, M. (1985) Family and school influences on behavioural development. *Journal of Child Psychology and Psychiatry, 26,* 349–368.

Rutter, M., Cox, A., Egert, S., Holbrook, D. & Everitt, B. (1981) Psychiatric interviewing techniques – IV. Experimental study: four contrasting styles. *British Journal of Psychiatry, 126,* 456–465.

Rutter, M., Izard, C. E. & Read, P. B. (eds) (1986) *Depression in Young People: Developmental and Clinical Perspectives.* New York, Guilford.

Rutter, M., Tizard, J. & Whitmore, K. (eds) (1970) *Education, Health and Behaviour.* London, Longman.

Sainsbury, C. P. Q., Gray, O. P. & Cleary, J. (1986) Care by parents of their children in hospital. *Archives of Disease in Childhood, 61,* 612–616.

Saylor, C. F., Pallmeyer, T. P., Finch, A. J., Eason, L., Treiber, F. & Folger, C. (1987) Predictors of psychological distress in hospitalised paediatric patients. *Journal of the American Academy of Child and Adolescent Psychiatry,* 232–236.

Schachar, R. (1991) Childhood hyperactivity. *Journal of Child Psychology and Psychiatry, 32,* 155–193.

Shah, N. (1981) Treatment of conductive deafness in children. In H. A. Beagley (ed.) *Audiology and Audiological Medicine, Vol. 2.* Oxford, Oxford University Press.

Shaw, J. (1990) Continence in cerebral palsy. *Health Visitor, 63,* 301–303.

Shearer, M. S. & Shearer, D. E. (1972) The Portage Project: a model for early childhood education. *Exceptional Child, 39,* 210–217.

Siegel, K., Mesagno, F. & Christ, G. (1990) A prevention program for bereaved children. *American Journal of Orthopsychiatry, 60,* 168–175.

Sloper, P., Knussen, C., Turner, S. & Cunningham, C. (1991) Factors related to stress and satisfaction with life in families of children with Down's syndrome. *Journal of Child Psychology and Psychiatry, 32,* 655–676.

Sluckin, W., Herbert, M. & Sluckin, A. (1983) *Maternal Bonding.* Oxford Blackwell.

Smith, J. (ed.) (1989) *Issues in Statementing Children with Emotional and Behavioural Problems: a Multi-disciplinary Approach.* Windsor, NFER-Nelson.

Snowling, M. J. (1991) Developmental reading disorders. *Journal of Child Psychology and Psychiatry, 32,* 49–79.

Spivak, G., Platt, J. J. & Shure, M. B. (1976) *The Problem Solving Approach to Adjustment.* San Francisco, Jossey-Bass.

Sroufe, L. A. (1985) Attachment classification from the perspective of infant caregiver relationships and infant temperament. *Child Development, 56,* 1–14.

Sroufe, L. A. & Fleeson, J. (1988) The coherence of family relationships. In R. Hinde & J. Stevenson (eds) *Relationships within Families.* Oxford, Oxford University Press.

Stacey, M., Dearden, R., Pull, R. & Robinson, D. (1970) *Hospitals, Children and their Families: a Pilot Study.* London, Routledge & Kegan Paul.

Stanley, L. (1980) Treatment of ritualistic behaviour in an eight-year-old girl by response prevention. *Journal of Child Psychology and Psychiatry, 21,* 85–90.

Stolberg, A. L. & Garrison, K. M. (1985) Evaluating a primary prevention program for children of divorce. *American Journal of Community Psychology, 13.*

Stratton, P. (1988) Understanding and treating child abuse in the family context: an overview. In K. Browne, C. Davies & P. Stratten (eds) *Early Prediction and Prevention of Child Abuse.* Chichester, Wiley.

Sylva, K. & Stein, A. (1990) Effects of hospitalisation on young children. *Newsletter of Association for Child Psychology and Psychiatry, 12,* 3–9.

Thibodeau, S. M. (1988) Sibling response to chronic illness: the role of the clinical nurse specialist. *Issues in Comprehensive Pediatric Nursing, 11,* 17–28.

Ungerer, J., Horagn, B., Chaitow, J. & Champion, G. B. (1988) Psychosocial functioning in children and young adults with juvenile arthritis. *Journal of Pediatrics, 81,* 195–202.

Van Eerdewegh, M., Bieri, M., Parilla, R. & Clayton, P. (1982) The bereaved child. *British Journal of Psychiatry, 140,* 23–29.

Van Hooft, S. (1990) Moral education for nursing decisions. *Journal of Advanced Nursing, 15,* 210–215.

Varni, J. W. & Wallander, J. L. (1988) Pediatric chronic disabilities: hemophilia and spina bifida as examples. In D. Routh (ed.) *Handbook of Pediatric Psychology.* New York, Guilford.

Vessey, J. A. (1988) Comparison of two teaching methods on children's knowledge of their internal bodies *Nursing Research, 37,* 262–267.

Vicary,. J. R. & Lerner, J. V. (1986) Parental attributes and adolescent drug use. *Journal of Adolescence, 9,* 115–122.

Wallerstein, J. (1991) The long-term effects of divorce on children: a review *Journal of the American Academy of Child and Adolescent Psychiatry, 30,* 349–359.

Wallerstein, J. & Kelly, J. (1980) *Surviving the Break-up: How Children and Parents Cope with Divorce.* New York, Basic Books.

Wassermand, G. A., Allen, R. & Solomon, C. R. (1985) At-risk toddlers and their mothers: the special case of physical handicap. *Child Development, 56,* 73–83.

White, M., Reynolds, B. & Evans, T. (1984) Handling of death in special care nurseries and parental grief. *British Medical Journal, 289,* 167–169.

White, R., Carr, P. and Lowe, N. (1990) *A Guide to the Children Act, 1989.* London, Butterworth.

Whitehead, N. (1989) Paediatrics and childhood cancer. In A. K. Broome (ed.) *Health Psychology: Processes and Applications.* London, Chapman & Hall.

WHO Europe (1981) Regional strategy for attaining health for all by the year 2000. EUR/RC 3018 rev. 1. Copenhagen, World Health Organization.

WHO Europe (1985) Targets for health for all. Copenhagen, World Health Organization.

Wolfer, J. A. & Visintainer, M. A. (1979) Prehospital psychological preparation for tonsillectomy patients: effects on children's and parent's adjustment. *Pediatrics, 64,* 646–655.

Woolley, H., Stein, A., Forrest, G. C. & Baum, J. D. (1989) Staff stress and job satisfaction at a children's hospice. *Archives of Diseases in Childhood, 64,* 114–118.

Zastowny, T. R., Kirschenbaum, D. S. & Meng, A. L. (1986) Coping skills training for children: effects on distress before, during and after hospitalisation for surgery. *Health Psychology, 5,* 231–247.

Zeitlin, S. & Williamson, G. G. (1990) Coping characteristics of disabled and non-disabled young children. *American Journal of Orthopsychiatry, 60,* 404–411.

Zurlinden, J. K. (1985) Minimising the impact of hospitalisation for children and their families. *American Journal of Maternal Child Nursing, 11,* 24–26.

Suggested answers to exercises

Exercise on p. 26

1. Toys in the cot.
2. Pictures and mobiles to look at.
3. A favourite toy or attachment object.
4. Mother by the bed.
5. Playleader or nurse for occupation and play.
6. Send him to the playroom. Why is he in his bed?
7. TV to watch.

Exercise on p. 62

There are many goals for establishing a parents' group each of which can be independently measured to gain an evaluation of its effectiveness.

1. To decrease incidence of common behaviour problems in young children e.g. sleeping, eating or general discipline.
2. To enhance child management skills.
3. To reduce the incidence of child abuse.
4. To enhance mothers' self esteem in coping with their children.
5. To reduce the incidence of maternal depression.
6. To reduce the level of social isolation.
7. To establish self support groups.
8. To identify the range and seriousness of pre-school behaviour problems in the community.

Outcome evaluation may depend on assessment before intervention compared to results after intervention or may just note parents' feelings about the value of the group. You could use any of the following:

1. Evaluation forms designed specifically for the project that parents fill in.
2. Published child behaviour checklists.
3. Published maternal mental health checklists.

232 Psychology and nursing children

4. Observations of mother–child interaction.
5. Reported incidences of child abuse.
6. Diaries of specific aspects of the child's behaviour e.g. sleep and eating diaries.
7. Interview of parents.

Exercise on p. 75

There is no simple answer to this exercise but certain principles are helpful and these different questions are useful at different times:

1. Mention positive qualities of the baby, to help the parents feel proud e.g. 'She has lovely hair', 'Isn't he sleeping beautifully?'
2. Make suppositions about how the parents might be feeling in order to draw out their reactions e.g. 'I guess this has been a tremendous shock.'
3. Enquire about their expectations and their knowledge e.g. 'Lots of parents worry about the possibility of something being wrong with their baby before it is born. Did you ever think about the possibility of this happening when you were pregnant? Do you know of anyone who has had a baby with any problems?'
4. Check that parents want the opportunity to talk about their baby e.g. 'I know this must be a very painful and worrying time for you, but if you would like to talk about what has happened, I am here to help. Would you like me to stay with you for a while?'
5. Try to elicit the parents' feelings and condone their expression of negative feelings e.g. 'I guess you must be feeling "why us?". Some parents feel very angry and want to blame someone.'
6. If parents start to cry then offer tissues quickly and wait quietly beside them until they want, or are able, to talk. Reassure them that it is right for them to cry.

Exercise on p. 105

Children show lots of different phobias:

Insects   – spiders, flying insects, wasps, bees
Animals – dogs, cats, snakes
Medical – hospitals, needles, doctors in white coats, oxygen masks
General – loud noises, darkness, thunder, heights, closed places, water
Specific – masks, clowns

Exercise on p. 116

Instructions to a mother about how to use a star chart for dry beds should include:

'Your child needs to be able to earn at least one star for a dry bed every few days, so he needs to show a little control first.

The star chart should be put up on the wall where your child can see and reach it.

The chart should be explained fully to your child so he knows what he has to do and what to expect.

If he has had a dry bed all night, he should receive a star to stick on his chart and be highly congratulated as soon as he gets up.

If he has a wet bed, just comment that tomorrow he could try to stay dry and then he could earn his star.

Under no circumstances should stars that have been awarded be taken away.

The main principle is that your child should realize how delighted you are with him, so when you give him a star he should be made to feel proud and good.'

Exercise on p. 117

If one child is hitting another child in the ward playroom:

1. You may need to prompt the mother to take control of her child and stop him hitting.
2. If she is unable or unwilling to control him you need to intervene and make it clear to both children that you expect no hitting in the playroom.
3. Watch the interaction and observe whether anything triggers the hitting e.g. wanting a toy held by the other child.
4. Teach the child another way of getting what he wants e.g. asking, bargaining, asking an adult for help, waiting until the other child has finished.
5. If he continues to hit then consider 'time out' of the playroom for five minutes and then allow him to return and try again.

Exercise on p. 120

To help a mother with her child's sleeping problems you could try the following:

1. Discuss whether the bottle feeding in the night is maintaining his waking and he is probably waking up for the bottle as a habit.
2. Recognize that he needs his bottle in order to fall asleep and has never learned to settle to sleep on his own.
3. Plan with the mother how to reduce the dependence on the bottle e.g. stop the bottle at night and offer a teacher beaker to reduce comfort sucking; or offer water in the bottle rather than preferred juice or milk; or gradually change the content of the bottle by adding more water; or gradually reduce the quantity offered in the bottle.
4. Plan with the mother how to reduce the child's physical dependence on her while falling asleep e.g. gradually reduce the amount of contact over successive nights while settling to sleep; or let the child fall asleep alone and do not go in even if he or she cries.

Exercise on p. 124

There are many different ways to design an observational chart for a child's behaviour. Here is one method, you may be able to think of several more:

Plan to observe the child every half hour for two minutes, code her behaviour, ask about any feelings of pain, and record who is with her at the time.

Behaviour code
Q = quiet, relaxed
A = active, moving around
E = eating
S = sleeping

Pain code
1 = no pain
2 = mild pain
3 = moderate pain
4 = severe pain

Time	Behaviour code	Pain code	Person present
7.00			
7.30			
8.00			
8.30			

Exercise on p. 130

There are a large number of problems some of which may be very
specific to individual families, so the nurse should find out from them
what is causing most difficulty.

Potential problems:

Asthma — management of asthma attacks at home, at night, in
school, at friends, while out shopping or on holiday
— avoidance of allergens e.g. extra house cleaning, change
of bedding, summer time pollen, cats and dogs
— exercising
— teaching self management to the child, compliance with
treatment
— coping with crises, use of medical services and hospitalization

Leukaemia — helping the child cope with invasive procedures and
treatment regime
— parents' and child's ability to cope with the effect of
treatment i.e. hair loss, nausea
— managing regular hospital visits, effect on family life,
financial costs
— explanation of the disease to the child
— planning for the future e.g. schools, holidays
— parental worry about the child's state

Exercise on p. 139

Target behaviour	Goal	Focus	Implementor
Physiotherapy	Prevent chest congestion	Child's illness	Mother
Go out for dinner	Normal marital relationships	Family system	Father
Ask for school work to be brought home	Maintain child's normal life	Social system	Mother
Family go swimming	Normal family activity	Family system	Sibling
Hospital visit	Check child's health	Child's illness	Mother

Exercise on p. 154

Questions that a nurse may ask to assess the child's prior experiences and current preferences include:

Is there anything he shouldn't eat because of religious beliefs or special diet? Does he eat ethnic, or English, food or both?

What religion is the family? Are there any special observances the nurses should know?

Does he understand English well? What language do you speak to him at home?

Has he slept away from home before? Does he have a special comforter for sleeping? Are there any special toys that he wants to take with him?

Does he know that he is coming to stay in hospital? Does he know why he is coming into hospital? How have you explained it to him?

Has he been in hospital before? If so, when, how long for, how many times? Has he had any invasive procedures before? How did he react?

Does he have pets at home; what are their names? Does he have any brothers and sisters? What are their names and how old are they?

Is there anything else that the parents feel the nurses should know about him?

Exercise on p. 165

Equipment that can be found in many ward play rooms include:

Creative materials for self expression – pencils and crayons, paints, Playdoh, collage work.

Fantasy play related to hospital – doctors and nurses kits including real and toy equipment; dressing up clothes; miniature hospital building with playpeople; dolls and teddies to demonstrate special procedures e.g. nasogastric tubes, gastrostomy tubes, Hickman's line, operation scars, plasters, drips.

Index

ABC chart 108–9
Abuse 35–9, 109
    non-accidental injury 35–7, 123
    psychological 35–7, 123
    screening for risk of 56–8
    sexual 35, 37–9, 123
Admission to hospital 146–9
    effects of 152–3
    helping the child 154
Adolescents 5, 33, 38, 43, 62, 79, 99,
        136, 144–5
    behaviour problems 102–3
    drug abuse 121
    dying 189–91
    emotional problems 104
    in hospital 159–62
Aggression 113, 116
Anorexia nervosa 103–4
Antisocial behaviour, management
        113–17
Anxiety 104–5
    anticipation 148–9, 172
    going into hospital 146–9
    management of 177–81
    parents 158–9
Assessment
    behaviour problems 55–6, 106–10
    developmental 55, 77, 107
    psychological 77–8, 60–1
Attachment 20–7
    babies 22–3
    parents 23–4
Attention deficit disorder 100
    management of 117–18
Autism 81–2

Behaviour problems in young children
        21, 33–4, 118–20
    see also Screening
Behaviour therapy, see Therapeutic
    approaches
Beliefs of children 3, 165–9, 183–6
Bell and pad 120
Bereavement 39–48, 196–7
    nurse intervention 45–8
Blindness, see Disability
Bonding 24
    see also Attachment

Care by parents 155–6
Cerebral palsy see Disability
Children Act (1989) 14–15, 51, 64,
        65–6, 67, 68, 71, 75–6
Child Development Centres 65
Child Guidance Units 64
Childhood Death Awareness Inventory 46
Childline 60
Child sexual abuse, see Abuse
Chronic disease 129–145
    effects on siblings 134–6
    family management style 130–40
Communication 7–9, 53–4
    hearing impaired 88–90
    non-verbal 7
Community health care 50–1, 53
    clinics 64
Compliance with treatment 3, 144
Compulsive rituals 122
Conduct problems 100
Consent for medical procedures 175–6
Consultation 10–12
Controlling pain 179
Conversion disorder 105
Coping
    nurse's role 142–4
    strategies 140, 150–1
    with chronic illness 140–3
    with chronic disorder 129–30
    with hospitalization 149–51
    with special needs 91–4
    with stress 170–1, 206–13
Counselling, see Therapeutic approaches
Cultural differences 7, 11, 30, 50–1,
        53–4, 56, 66, 74, 130–2, 148

Day care 27, 68, 69
Deafness see Disability
Death 39–48
    after death 196
    child's concept of 39–41, 183–6
    of parent 42–3
    of sibling 43–4
    religion 41–2
    see also Bereavement
Depression
    childhood 105
    management of 123–4
    maternal 28–9

Diabetes   142–4
Disability
   cerebral palsy   84, 86
   diagnosis   71–5
   hearing impairment   88–90
   physical   83–7
   sensory   87–90, 107–8
   spina bifida   84, 96
   visual   87–8
Disintegrative psychosis   106, 124
Distraction   178, 179
Divorce   19, 31–5, 129
Downs syndrome   79–81, 91–5
Drug abuse   102–3
   management of   121
Dying
   adolescent   189–91
   at home   193–4
   children   186–9
   farewells   192–3
   in hospital   194–6
   parents of   191–2
Dyslexia   83

Eating problems – young children
   118–19
Education
   Education Act (1981)   76–7
   Education service   68–9
   Education welfare service   69
   in hospital   163–5
Emotions   9, 71, 104–5, 134–6
Encopresis   101
   management of   120–1
Enuresis   100–1
   management of   120
Ethics   216–19

Facial expression   7, 53
Family centres   63
Family
   relationships   5
   breakdown   31–4
Family therapy, *see* Therapeutic approaches
Fears   122
Freedom   217

Groups
   community   60–4
   ethnic   63–4
   parents   60–1, 63
   play   63
   self-help   62
   support   62–3
   therapy   112
   voluntary   62
Guided imagery   177–8

Health education   2
Health promotion   52

Hospice   194
Hospitalization   146–51
Hyperactivity   100
   behavioural management   117
   dietary management   117–18
Hypnotherapy   112, 178

Illness
   child's understanding   165–9
   socio-economic factors   50–1
   psychological factors   60
Information giving   12, 14
Interview technique   106

Language development   12, 77, 81, 96
Learning difficulties   76–81
   mild   82–3
   severe   77–9
   specific   83
Long-stay hospitalization   162–3

Makaton   89–90
Maternal depression, *see* Depression
Maternal deprivation   26–7
   see also Attachment
Mourning   44–5

Obsessional thoughts   122

Pain
   concept of   177
   emergencies   180–1
   management of   177–81
   reporting of   3
Parenting   27–8
   breakdown   35
Parents on the ward   155–8
Partnership with parents   9–10, 14–15
Patients' rights   216, 218
Pharmacotherapy, *see* Therapeutic
   approaches
Phobias   122
Play
   groups   63
   in hospital   163–5, 171, 173
   medically related   3
Portage   81
Positive reinforcement   115–16
Preparation
   for hospitalization   146–51
   for procedures   171–5
Pre-school behaviour problems   100
Prevention   58–60
   primary   58–9
   secondary   59–60
Psychosomatic disorders   123
Psychotherapy   112
Punishment   35

Questionnaires
  Behaviour Checklist 55–6
  Behaviour Screening Questionnaire
    55
  Children's Behaviour Checklist 55
  Child Death Awareness Inventory
    46–8
  General Health Questionnaire 56, 204
  Pre-school Behaviour Questionnaire
    55
  Ways of Coping Scale 208
Questioning
  directive 8
  non-directive 8

Relationships
  family 5, 19, 53, 73, 91, 130
  parent–child 28–9, 94, 137, 144, 158
  therapeutic 7, 14
Relaxation exercises 150, 178
Religion
  death 41–2
Residential care 67

Safety 2
Schizophrenia, childhood 105–6, 124
School refusal 122
Schools Psychological Service 69
Screening
  abuse 56–8
  behaviour problems 54–6
  developmental and language problems
    55
Self help, *see* Groups
Separation
  marital 31–5
  on the ward 158
  parent–child 23, 24–5
Sexual abuse, *see* Abuse
Single parents 19, 31
Sleep problems 118–19
Social class 29–30, 50–1
Social Services 65–8

Social stress 29–30
Social support 138–9, 140
Special needs
  families 71, 91–5
  nurse's role 95–6
Spina bifida, *see* Disability
Star charts 115–16, 119, 120
Stress
  causes of 202–6
  coping with 150–1, 170–1, 206–13
  effect of 201
Stressful procedures 153
Suggestion in pain relief 179–80
Suicide 105, 124
Symptoms, reporting 3
Systematic desensitisation 122

Therapeutic approaches 111–13
  behaviour therapy 111–12, 113–16,
    117–21, 123
  cognitive/behaviour therapy 117
  counselling 112
  family therapy 111, 121, 136–8
  group therapy 112
  hypnotherapy 112, 178
  individual therapy 112
  pharmacotherapy 113
Therapeutic relationship 6
Time out 114
Toilet training 119, 120
Treatment compliance 3, 144–5
Trust 216–17

Unconditional positive regard 6

Visiting in hospital 155
Voluntary groups 62
  see also Groups
Voluntary organisations 69

World Health Organisation 51–2
Working with parents 9, 11